"Dr. Noel Lloyd knocks it out of the park with *The Chiropractor's Guide*! I wish I would've had this information when I began practice. Would've made things easier, less stressful, and more profitable... There are so many great ideas, resources, protocols and scripts in Dr. Noel's book. If you're a chiropractor interested in making a bigger impact and generating dramatically more practice revenue, read this immediately."

—*Matthew Loop, author of* Social
Media Made Me Rich

"Bravo! Noel Lloyd has provided the definitive answer to the question, 'How do I get more new patients?' Crisp writing. Zero fluff. Practical, immediately-usable ideas that capture the head, heart and hands required to make a ruckus and help a lot of people. Makes me wish I was a chiropractor!"

—*William D. Esteb, founder and
president of Patient Media, Inc.*

"Over the nearly fifty years of my chiropractic life I have met all kinds of chiropractors. I have always been drawn to passionate, hard-working, get-the-job done kind of DCs. Reading Noel's book was like have an extended conversation with all of them at once! This is a complete and concise read for any DC, from a recent graduate to the seasoned gray hair. There are no wasted words, no unnecessary prose, just well organized, logically presented and easily absorbed counsel for anyone wishing to help patients, have fun, and make money in practice as a chiropractor! Anyone who follows the advice offered in this guide will be successful, period."

—*Gerard Clum, President Emeritus,
Life Chiropractic College West*

The Chiropractor's Guide

56 Proven Ways to Help More People,
Have More Fun, and Make More Money

By Noel Lloyd, DC

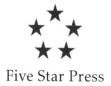

Five Star Press

The Chiropractor's Guide
© 2016 Noel Lloyd

For more information about this book or the author, visit
http://www.myfivestar.com

ISBN 978-0-9982657-0-4
eISBN 978-0-9982657-1-1

First edition 2016
Printed in the United States of America

This book is designed to provide information and motivation. The information provided within this book is for general informational purposes only, and no warranties or guarantees are expressed or implied for an individual reader's outcome. While every example and story is true, some names and identifying details have been changed to protect the privacy of individuals.

Cover design by Tiger Bright Studios
Interior design and production by Sharper Words, LLC

For my wife, Kate

Contents

Introduction

Late one night I was driving back to Seattle with three of my associates. We'd spent the day visiting a successful chiropractor, and we were talking about what we'd observed about chiropractic and practice success.

"It all boils down to helping a lot of people, having a lot of fun, and making a lot of money," I said, articulating for the first time what I now call the Tri-Fold Objective.

"People first, fun second, and money last, but chiropractors have the unique opportunity to do all three in a wonderful mix."

Ever since that day, I have made this the question that guides my practice: "How does this help us help more people, have more fun, and make more money?" I've measured everything I do in business against these three simple goals. They have guided me as I built and sold ten successful clinics and developed dozens of great associates, and as I now run two successful practice management companies.

And now I want to share them with you. In this book, I've collected my cream-of-the-crop tips and advice to guide your chiro-

practic practice to success, filtered through the Tri-Fold Objective
and tested for tens of thousands of hours over many decades.

There are many ideas that didn't make the cut for this book.
Over the years, I've tried hundreds of things that did not work. I've
rejected fads that promised easy money because I wasn't convinced
they would help people. I've thought long and hard about how
to make everything that happens in my offices as much fun as
possible, and I've streamlined the business part of the practice to
consistently return a better profit.

What you'll find here are the strategies, programs, and procedures I've polished into systems that work. Thousands of successful chiropractic practices around the world are using my methods
to build the practices of their dreams, and their successes are the
living proof that the Tri-Fold Objective works.

First, let's help a lot of people.

As chiropractors, we have the opportunity to help people in a
way no other doctor can—through innate healing. The chiropractor
who comprehends and witnesses that power knows they have a
sacred mission to get this message and care to as many people as
possible.

Many of us chose chiropractic because of what chiropractic
did for us personally. I know that's the case for me—my life was
changed forever by a chiropractic adjustment over sixty years ago.
It has always been my goal to give that same experience to others.
Helping others validates our experience, our belief in, and our
commitment to chiropractic.

How many times have you listened to stories of failed medical
treatments, near-death experiences because of drug reactions, and
people with chronic pain who are told they'll just have to "learn to
live with it"? Thankfully, for them and us, there is a better way.

You know it when you see the thankful face of a former migraine sufferer who says, "It's been seven months without a migraine, Doctor. I can't thank you enough."

Or when you see the shy smile of the twelve-year-old boy who used to wet the bed every night. "Over a hundred days with no accidents, Doctor, and I went on my first ever sleepover last weekend with no problem. Thanks."

Or when you hold a brand new baby born to a woman who'd been infertile for eight years due to a lumbar subluxation you found and corrected.

I could list chiropractic miracles forever, because new ones are created faster than I can write, and this is why we're here.

By helping people first, we align our heads and hearts with the best motives of loving service. Helping people puts us into the role of caregiver, giving the best we have, co-laboring with the healing source of life that built not only our bodies but also the entire universe—what we chiropractors know as Innate and Universal Intelligence.

The best chiropractors I know feel that it is their mission to help as many people as possible. They're committed to growing busy practices, where the only limitations are the requirements of their chosen technique.

They know that taking care of more patients can give a committed chiropractor more energy than it requires. I remember the Fridays I left the office on an emotional "high" after a week filled to the brim with hours of co-laboring with the power that made the universe. The days flew by as my staff, associates, and I committed ourselves fully to the moment, practicing the art of chiropractic on patients with seemingly magical results.

That's why the first priority is always to help more people. I'll show you how to do that by establishing a practice you'll be proud to call your own, because it's appealing to visitors and connected to the community.

Next, let's have more fun.

Who wouldn't love to have more fun? Everyone wants to enjoy their work. It's natural to want to have a practice you can look forward to—a practice that feels like a hobby or a game we can't wait to play because it's just plain fun.

Well, you can. You can have so much fun in your chiropractic practice that you'd be hard-pressed to think of anywhere you'd rather be.

Some might think that *real* fun is living with no responsibilities and millions of dollars in the bank. But every day the news tells us about the crumbling lives of those who had those privileges and clearly weren't having much fun.

It's fun to be needed, to serve with clear purpose and motives, and to work shoulder to shoulder with a team of people you respect, in service to others.

It's fun to be in the moment—what some of us call present-time consciousness—with your patients, guided by a strong chiropractic philosophy and focused on an excellent adjustment, confident that the other pieces of your practice are functioning well without your micromanagement.

When you're focused, confident, and doing great work, you'll get into an enjoyable rhythm where you are growing and thriving personally, as well as professionally. Your decisions will become intuitive, decisive, and compassionate. You'll move into what I call the "zone."

Picture a top-performing sports team, where the players are all trained to do their positions with precision and practiced coordination. All of their work and preparation is worth it on game day, when the victory is won. That's the type of fun I'm talking about.

Have you ever had the experience of using great tools in the kitchen or great skis on the mountain—or of driving a well-tuned sports car that seemed to anticipate your unspoken desire and move effortlessly through the corners? That's the fun that I want to show you how to have.

Now, let's also make more money.

I debated putting "make more money" in this book title for a long time. I was worried that someone might misunderstand my purpose or think I want to teach chiropractors how to take advantage of their patients.

But let's be real. Regardless of our profession, we want be paid well for the work we do. And a successful, fun practice that helps people also makes money.

Here's my promise: you can provide the highest quality chiropractic care, with incredible customer service that everyone is proud of and enjoys, while charging reasonable prices—never overcharging or doing one more adjustment than is necessary—and still make great money.

You can have a sleek and streamlined business system that runs like a Swiss watch, serving up that beautiful chiropractic care, and also supports your financial goals—whether that's paying off school loans, getting out of all debt, buying a nice house and car, sending the kids to school, or saving for retirement. You can even finally take those memorable vacations you've been dreaming about. I'll show you how to set up your practice so that you're making money even when you're out of the office.

Finally, let's put it all together.

For decades, the Tri-Fold Objective of helping more people, having more fun, and making more money has guided the decisions I make in both my personal chiropractic practices, Sound Chiropractic Centers, and my management service for chiropractors, Five Star Management.

If it doesn't truly help people, if we can't be proud of it, if we wouldn't recommend it to our families, we don't do it, and I don't ask my clients to do it.

If it isn't fun, we'll tweak it and train for it until it is, or we'll scrap it and start over.

And if it doesn't support the business by making money, we don't do it. That's how we keep going so that we can help more people and have more fun. The great little bakery or dry cleaner whose business model didn't work (didn't make money) isn't there next year.

The Chiropractor's Guide will show you how to implement these same three ideas.

Start by picturing your practice. Your parking lot is full, and your reception area is comfortably crowded. Your front desk CA is answering phones, smiling, and laughing with patients who are thrilled to be there. Your adjusting area is busy, and you and your associates are moving smoothly and confidently from patient to patient. It's been an extra busy and satisfying day.

At 4:30 p.m., your senior associate steps up and says, "I'll take over the rest of your patients, Doc. You've got a plane to catch."

He smiles as he hands you your keys and phone. You smile back as your lead CA tells you, "Don't even think of us. You've earned this vacation. We've got it. You have fun."

In that instant, you know they really do "have it," and the patients are in excellent hands. As you drive home to pick up your family for a much-anticipated holiday, you realize how blessed you are to be a chiropractor. You love helping people, your team makes your job fun, and you make a great living.

That's what *The Chiropractor's Guide* is all about.

Are you ready?

Part One

Help More People

Taking Care of Your Patients

1

The Thirteen Keys to Your Dream Practice

Fact: Every chiropractor worth their salt wants a busy, thriving practice. We feel our best when we're helping lots of people, having tons of fun, and making a good living.

Fact: The stakes are high. Failures are common, and practices that are new and small are most vulnerable. All the time and money you put into your education, plus your practice start-up costs and your future, are riding on how well you quickly build a strong, successful practice.

Fact: Most doctors will never realize the dreams that attracted them to chiropractic because they never got the training or mentoring they needed to break out of mediocrity and into success.

This book changes that.

While everything in this book is written to help you, this first chapter could be the most important guidance you've ever read. It contains the thirteen keys to your dream practice—selected success concepts, ideas, strategies, and tips for building a great practice in less time than you ever thought possible. I'll unpack these ideas in subsequent chapters, as well as offer additional tips and advice learned through experience. But this chapter outlines the bottom line, and I'm giving it to you right up front.

Key #1: The Big Decision

This is a big one, so please read it carefully. I'm asking you to make the most important decision you can make to build your dream practice. In fact, very few doctors ever get there without making this decision.

I'm asking you to decide to love the process. Whatever it takes to build your dream practice, decide to love it.

I'm asking you to love it all: the struggles, the journeys, the work, the battles, the growth, the character building, the skill acquisition, and the endurance—as well as the wins, the accomplishments, and the people you will help along the way. Decide NOW that you'll love it.

This is what all successful people learn to do.

What you actually learn to love is the challenge of fighting and winning. And there's no way to win without this type of commitment.

The guy who was once overweight and now has six-pack abs didn't wake up one day to find a magically sleek midriff. He certainly didn't buy one of those crazy gimmick ab machines that promises to work if he does sit-ups for "ten minutes a day, three times a week."

No, Mr. Abs decided he would do whatever it took, and he committed to (fell in love with) the process. In his case, that was probably a low-fat diet and a zillion ab crunches of every description, every day.

One committed weight lifter I know put it this way: "I now really love doing what I once really hated, and that's exercise."

[Handwritten margin notes: "Someone else's goals", "job", "dream practice = your own goals"]

Every person who has built a dream practice in fewer than ninety days (or 180 days) worked ~~like crazy,~~ but they also never let it become drudgery, and it never felt like a job. A job is something you do for someone else's goals. Building your dream practice is something you do for your own goals.

When you fall in love with the process, it becomes your mission and your passion. You love what you're creating, because you made the decision to do whatever it took.

The decision comes first, so make that decision now. There is no real success without it.

Key #2: Lots and Lots of New Patients

If the first key (choosing to love the process) is the most important attitude, the second key is the most important action/skill set.

Learn how to produce new patients—lots and lots of new patients.

Every doctor who has a dream practice knows that getting new patients is key. No matter how well you set that atlas or adjust that lumbar, you have to know how to get new patients.

This is the truth: I've known great DCs who, sadly, now do other work because they couldn't market chiropractic, and I also know mediocre docs who have large practices because they have some natural marketing talent or learned some skills. You can't do anything about your gene pool, but 99 percent of you can acquire the skills needed to produce new patients…if you fall in love with the process.

Let me tell you just a few real-life stories about dream practice doctors. You'll get the idea.

I opened a clinic in a mall. We did spinal screenings that produced 161 new patients the first month. We hit 206 visits in our seventh week.

I showed a client how to do this same type of opening, and he set up a screening that got *more than 110 new patients the first month and 231 visits his fourth week*. All of this happened in a brand new practice.

Another client spent two days with me designing a marketing plan for the practice that he was opening in two months. After the opening, we spoke every week, and he reported on his marketing responsibilities: networking, screenings, business contacts, and professional contacts. This guy was so excited that every day he had a new story. He hit *more than 200 visits in less than 150 days*. He says that the whole process was fun, scary, and exciting, all at the same time.

Remember the part about learning to love the process?

Several new DC graduates have done apprenticeships with my clients using the Win-Win Associate Development systems, which I'll describe later in the book. They launched their own practices by starting business-to-business networking thirty days prior to opening. They followed that by offering screenings at festivals, block parties, community fairs, health fairs, and health clubs. Additionally, they met every dentist, general practitioner, attorney, and business owner in town. (If your clinic is still under construction, you have the time to do these things. If you're already in practice, you can set aside three to seven hours per week to be your own marketing director.)

Several clients managed to do well with newspaper advertising and literally produced so many new patients that they had people standing in a line across the back of the reception area filling out their paperwork. In one of my offices, we had twenty-two new patients in one day. It was hard work and a bit chaotic, of course, but very exciting! And think of all the people who heard the whole chiropractic story for the very first time at that standing-room-only New Patient Orientation class.

Maybe that doesn't sound ideal, but it's a better problem than wondering if your phone has been disconnected or someone has locked your front door.

If I get to choose my problems, give me that terrible "too many new patients" problem any day.

Every dream practice I've coached has a diversified marketing strategy where the doctor works at least three external marketing programs and three internal marketing programs simultaneously. One or two of those programs inevitably takes off like a rocket, a couple are steady and worth the effort, and some just don't fly and need to be swapped out.

Get too many new patients, and all your "problems" will be fun and exciting. Get too few new patients, and nothing is fun or exciting.

Key #3: A Strong Day One

How many times have you heard "You never get a second chance at a first impression?" Right or wrong, a patient's first impression of you is what they'll use to judge you. Why not make it a great one? *for any interaction*

What impresses a new patient? What do they want from a new doctor? More than fancy surroundings, every patient wants to be cared for and led.

"If you don't care about me (put my interest above your own) I won't trust you. If you can't lead me, you're irrelevant." *TRUST*

Another axiom that applies here is that "people believe the message only after they believe the messenger." With this in mind, you need to have a strong (impressive) first day for new patients. *have to build it w/ confidence*

Here are some key points for Day One:

Polish up your office. Make sure it's clean, vacuumed, and dusted and has a nice fragrance. Have upbeat music playing. Get

People late having their name Remembered

NAMES

rid of the dead plant and the clutter. Display chiropractic educational material on plasma screens and in testimony books. Paint one wall in the reception area a fresh new accent color. Then ask an honest friend to evaluate the office. Make more changes if needed.

Polish up your CA. Role-play with your CA to lock in a cheerful greeting for new patients when they enter your office. There's nothing more impressive than a friendly and enthusiastic CA who stands, smiles, and says, "You must be Mrs. Carlson. My name is Mandy. Welcome to our office."

Keep the initial paperwork to a minimum. People want to see the doctor ASAP. Trim their paperwork time to no more than ten minutes.

Practice your own clinical skills. Saying the right thing at the right time is important. Role-play and practice the best ways to take a history. Your exam process will vary according to philosophy and technique, but make sure you can do yours with skill and confidence.

if needed ← **When appropriate, insist on X-rays or other scans.**

Give each new patient a home care sheet. This will launch your new patient's care and help them feel better.

Schedule a report of findings (ROF) for the next day. Take the time to analyze your patient's history, exam, and X-rays (when indicated) before you outline a care plan and start adjusting. The best clinical approach educates your patient on chiropractic, their specific problem, and your solution.

Key #4: A Strong Day Two

TRUST

Good patient relationships are crafted or crushed in the first two days.

A strong Day One gives you the clinical information you need and the patient the confidence that they're in the right hands. A strong Day Two can establish a doctor-patient relationship that lasts for a lifetime.

The following are important points to remember for a strong Day Two:

Tell all staff members to learn each new patient's name on Day One and be able to greet the patient by name on Day Two. This may seem trivial, but I assure you, it isn't. I have done more than a dozen patient focus groups, and this is the only thing common to all the groups: *Everyone liked being remembered by name.* → See?

Don't make your patients wait. It may sound too simple, but patients shouldn't wait for more than five minutes. It's common

Learn how to give a good report of findings. There are so few curtesy home runs in practice, but the ROF, when done well, definitely qualifies.

Your report of findings explains:
- How chiropractic works
- The seriousness of the patient's subluxation
- Your best care recommendations for their case

When making care recommendations, outline the care you truly think the patient needs. Don't under-recommend care. or over → Trust

You're now ready to start your patient's care. A good Day Two also teaches each patient how to be a successful patient in your office. I call this our office orientation.

By the end of Day Two, your new patient should know what to expect from their chiropractic care over the next few days, have their appointments scheduled in advance, and have had a financial consultation that puts their mind at rest regarding paying for their care.

They should feel comfortable with the process even if they are still in pain.

At the end of clinic hours, call all of your Day Two or first adjustments to make sure they are doing well. Your patients will appreciate the care and attention to detail.

Key # 5: Visit a Dream Practice Model

A picture is worth a thousand words. Never is that more true than the picture of the practice you would like to have. Make it a goal to find and visit the type of practice you want to grow: a place where they help a lot of people, have a lot of fun, and are financially successful. Try to see, hear, smell, touch, and even taste it. This will sharpen your vision/goals, and affirmations for where you want to end up.

Years ago, before I was a consultant, I flew to the San Francisco Bay area and just dropped in on the three biggest chiropractic practices in the country. I wanted to watch those practices quietly, from the shadows. Surprisingly, what I got instead was the red carpet treatment. They each showed me everything in their practice. I experienced a huge increase that year in my own practice due to having a much clearer vision.

I learned that day that when it's working correctly, successful doctors love to show others what they've learned and how beautiful their practices are.

Find out who uses your chiropractic technique and sees the patient volume you want to see. I showed up unannounced, but today that's too risky and too brash. Instead, give the doctor a call, and ask if you can visit their practice to watch for a couple of their busy hours. Offer to take them out to lunch or dinner and pick their brain.

Even if it's a four-hour drive, or a long train ride, or a flight away, the experience will be worth it. Can you take a three-day road trip to see three or four practices? You'll never be the same. I promise.

Key #6: Don't Go It Alone!

I bet you watched at least some of the recent Olympic Games, where world records went tumbling and new records were set.

The experts will debate what makes an Olympic athlete unique, but I know at least one thing they have in common with each other that's different from most of us: they each have a coach. They also have training partners. Olympic-caliber athletes are typically the best in the world, but they also know the power of staying in relationship with those who can help get them to where they want to go.

Birds of a feather do flock together.

Key #7: A New Practice Is Like a New Baby

A well-established practice has a strength and momentum that a new practice doesn't have. *Any Goal*

Building your dream practice is like caring for a new baby. A new practice needs constant care and attention. That's not unique to chiropractic practices—every new business needs that type of care. It's why new parents and new business owners have to put in all the overtime. You're always feeding, tending, and changing. *Remember*

Good doctors building their dream practice will do whatever is necessary to make sure their baby thrives. Please don't confuse this with a job. Your kids may be work, but they aren't a job, and neither is your dream practice. *dream → practice*

You would not take a vacation and leave the baby at home. A new practice can't take that much neglect either. If you've been working like crazy to get the practice going and build momentum, and you've finally added one hundred visits to your weekly volume, this is not the time to overindulge in time off and holidays. This is the time to come in early, stay late, and work through lunch when needed. *job*

Your first real holiday may not come for over a year in a new practice, and when it does, it may be just four days long. And even then, it's smart to hire a babysitter (a locum). Take Thursday through Sunday off for yourself, but hire a relief doctor for Friday afternoon, and book every patient in the shortest amount of time possible when you return. *Keep it Steady*

Key #8: Keep Up the Marketing

This happens almost every time: a DC thinks that when their initial marketing push to launch a new clinic or double an existing practice ends, that's the end of their marketing efforts. But that's just the wrong way to think about it.

Where did all of your new patients come from initially? Marketing, right? Exactly, and that's where they will come from for quite a while. If you quit marketing, then you stop doing what made you successful, and things will crash. This isn't rocket science, but it seems to elude quite a few docs. The temptation to quit marketing too soon is almost irresistible.

That doesn't mean you won't get referrals. You will. But here's what I tell my associates: we will be doing some type of external marketing every day, even if it's only an hour. We will do that for days, weeks, and months, until we're so busy we can't leave the patients in the clinic to go meet more. Then we'll train assistants to do our marketing.

Remember, not enough new patients is the number one problem in chiropractic practices today. Learning how to attract new patients is the most valuable practice-building skill you can develop. Once you start the marketing engine, keep it going. I can't tell you how many doctors have lamented cutting back, so keep up the marketing.

Key #9: Watch Your Time

This key requires a short setup, but it's worth it, so here goes: Your clinic is like a computer. The facilities and equipment are the hardware, and the systems you use to take care of patients constitute the operating system—like a computer uses Windows 7 or Mac OS X. Your clinic's operating system will make seeing a high patient volume either smooth and easy, or rough and clumsy.

Since they don't teach "clinic operating system" in school, you learn it on your own when you start practicing. But there's a problem—that's also the time when you aren't very busy, and consequently, you could also be a little lonely. During this time, efficiency has little value.

With those bad habits in place, a clinic ends up topping out at 100, 80, even as few as 60 visits a week. The doctors tell us that everything feels as if they are running through wet concrete, and they are exhausted at the end of the week.

On the other hand, a doctor who has a good clinic operating system can see many times that number of patients in a relaxed manner.

So how do you install a new and more efficient clinic operating system?

It starts with watching your time. How long does it take to adjust your spouse? Probably not long. Why should it take longer to adjust other patients? I suggest you ask your CA to time you—not so you try to break any speed records, but so you know how much time you take with new patients, regular adjustments, re-examinations, re-X-rays, re-evaluations and re-reports. You're going to be surprised. If you're like most doctors, your perception of time and the real time it takes will be very different.

One way to win back time is to *just focus on chiropractic when you're with your patients*. Patients want to hear about themselves,

People

their care, and chiropractic. I'll talk about chiropractic philosophy, technique, testimonies, great moments, and great patients. But if they try to drag me into a personal conversation, or talk about rugby or football, I resist the temptation. Patients are much happier with doctors who focus on chiropractic.

You're either training your patients to burn up a lot of your emotional energy, or you're training them to focus on what gives both of you energy: chiropractic. → love the process

Do what the real pros do consistently: practice your procedures (Day One and Two, etc.) away from the practice, for critique and time. Get together with your DC buddy from across town and take them through a Day One. See how long it takes, and ask for their critique. Next week, do Day Two.

Key #10: Checklists and Templates

In order to keep things running smoothly and keep things as simple as possible, doctors who have dream practices create checklists and templates for each procedure.

Regrettably, many doctors never do the same thing the same way twice. That creates stress, producing rethinking and second guessing. No one knows what's going on from visit to visit when the doctor makes it up as they go along. That's inefficient and exhausting. YES!!

The dream practice way is to use checklists and templates: Do each procedure the right way every time, write it down the way you want it done, and practice.

A routine visit using checklists and templates may look like the following:

- CA(s) and DC(s) cheerfully greet the patient by their first name when the patient enters the clinic.

People love consistency

- Patient signs in, makes a payment, confirms their next appointment, and is informed about an upcoming reexam, all by the front desk CA.
- Patient escorts themselves back to the adjustment room or hot seats.
- Patient marks a subjective code sheet showing how they are responding to care.
- Patient moves to the adjusting table, completes preadjustment exercises, and studies the patient education for that day.
- Doctor greets the prepared patient and does an expert precheck, adjustment, postcheck, chiropractic education, and chart note, then releases the patient to their next step.
- Patient goes to therapy or rest (when indicated) or is released.
- Patient's super-low-stress checkout is reduced to a wave as they leave the clinic and a "Good-bye, Anita. See you Wednesday!"

This well-choreographed "dance" has several steps and needs a choreographer. Once you know what you want to see (what you want done) in your office, the next step is to make a checklist of each desired dance step and template those steps into a sequence.

You can create a checklist and template for every job description, every procedure, and every patient connection. Then, instead of accidental greatness, you have a chance at purposeful perfection.

When you use checklists and templates you're working with the same concepts as recipes and formulas. If you want a great cake, follow a great recipe.

Does this sound too mechanical for you? It's the opposite. Once you know the dance steps, you teach your partners (associates, CAs, and patients), and then you all forget the mechanics and are free to just focus on chiropractic, the patient, and the moment.

Net result: high-volume, low-stress, easy-to-use, day-to-day clinic procedures.

Key #11: Specialize in Excellent Customer Service

Think about the places where you "do business" again and again: the coffee shop, dry cleaner, restaurant, you name it. I'm betting you're treated well, and there are few frustrations. That's good customer service.

Make or break

Combine that thought with the fact that 67 percent of the people who decide never to frequent a business again do so because of poor customer service, and you see the need to work on great customer service.

Here's my short list of customer service points to consider:

- An office presentation that's not fancy but is clean, cheerful, and upbeat. People relate to their environments with all five senses, so freshen the paint, vacuum, dust, wash the windows, clean the bathroom, empty the trash, use scented candles, play appropriate upbeat music, and keep the temperature just right.
- Staff presentation that begins with clean uniforms or appropriate clothing, as well as practiced, enthusiastic greetings, quickly remembering the patient's name.
- Convenient office hours that serve the community and make it easy to get care and refer friends.
- Staff who are quick to listen to patient problems and to say, "That's terrible! Let me get that fixed right away." This is the opposite response of the "tough luck" shrug. Staff should always take the patient's side in their problem and find a solution that puts us all on the same side. Do not make it "us against them."
- A commitment to follow up and get back to patients with details and answers to their questions. This often is a billing

issue and can be handled with prompt phone calls or Post-it notes attached to their files.

- Care and respect for the patient's time. Don't make them wait if at all possible, but if it happens, apologize for the inconvenience. How personal is acceptable? pg. 14
- Making personal phone calls. If a patient is going through a "rough patch," a phone call from the doctor expressing your personal concern is the very picture of customer service.

I have learned plenty more tips, both big and small, that make a huge difference in how patients bond to their doctors, offices, and chiropractic in general. Becoming a student of customer service has helped me experience huge benefits.

Key #12: Mentor Your Associate

When you've gone through this process of building your own dream practice, you will have acquired extremely valuable skills and information. Plus, you will need help taking care of all these lovely patients. That's when you want to find an associate to train and mentor.

Even though one chiropractor can see hundreds of visits a week, when you build a dream practice, you can multiply your efforts even more by finding, hiring, and developing top-notch associates. There are hundreds of doctors who would like to be mentored in just this type of associateship.

Here's how I like to think about it:

My purpose as a chiropractor is to teach people about innate intelligence and the healing power that is within the body. I do that by finding people who need chiropractic care and introducing them to the beautiful science, art, and philosophy of chiropractic, packaged in a wonderful little practice/business that runs like a Swiss watch.

As an analogy, chiropractic is like fine wine. The practice or business is the carefully crafted stemware. Without the goblet, the wine is just a mess on the tablecloth. Similarly, without the carefully crafted business systems that market, process, care for, and collect from those patients, we're out of business.

A successful chiropractor seeks to pass the philosophical, clinical, and business concepts on to associates. I want to build in others a love for people, chiropractic, and a keen appreciation for a very specialized business that is a practice.

I've done this for dozens of associates, and ten times I've launched my associates into their own practices, giving them the chance to own and prosper in their own clinics. I've made good money in this process, but it hasn't been just about the money.

A huge part of the payoff is that I became a teacher, mentor, coach, player, conductor, and producer. I passed on the knowledge to someone else and helped their journey.

Key #13: Never Give Up

Sheer determination is worth more than everything else. I love the Sir Winston Churchill quote, "Never, never, never, never give up."

He nailed it down even tighter when he said, "Never give in, never give in, never, never, never, never—in nothing, great or small, large or petty—never give in except to convictions of honor and good sense."

I believe that chiropractic and your dream practice are large, wonderful, and worthwhile. They are neither small nor petty. They are worth all you can give them.

2

Love and Lead

I'm grateful to have the best vantage point in chiropractic—my consulting chair. On a daily basis, I help some of the best doctors on the planet serve their communities, build spectacular practices, reach their goals, and realize long-cherished dreams. It's always rewarding, and from time to time, the clarity that comes from seeing so many practices is breathtaking.

Let me give you an example. Everyone wants great patient retention, but few understand what the best patient retention is made of.

Strong philosophy? Essential. Good procedures? Without a doubt. But the most important factors of patient retention are what I call "love and lead."

I've seen this again and again. The doctors with the best patient visit average (PVA) really love their patients and are not afraid to lead them—even when those actions are costly.

What do I mean by "loving" the patient? Quite simply, putting their best interests first, ahead of your own. Going out of your way to serve them. Think how you would want your family cared

19

for. That's what love looks like. It isn't sentimental, but it does consider the thoughts and feelings of other individuals.

For love to really be tested, it has to be inconvenienced. For doctors, that means caring enough to spend time and money to be certified in your technique. Coming in early or staying late for someone who was stuck shows you are willing to be inconvenienced. That's usable and practical love.

What do I mean by "leading" the patient? Being courageous enough to teach them about chiropractic, even if you might be misunderstood. Let the strength of your convictions show as you outline the required care and gently but firmly encourage your patient to do whatever the right thing is—whether it's keeping their appointments, doing their exercises, or not ruining their adjustments. Leadership includes standing with people where they are, focusing on their best future, and asking them to follow you to a healthier place.

If you love me but can't lead me, you're irrelevant. If you lead me but don't love me, I don't trust you.

Over time, patients and entire communities will learn whether you can love and lead, and when they do, they will gladly follow you to their best health decisions and stay with you and chiropractic for a lifetime.

3

How to Help Your Ideal Patient Find You

Imagine you're at the front desk looking at the schedule as a smile creeps across your face. Row after row, name after name, hour after hour, you're about to be blessed with an entire day of ideal patients. "Every day should be like this," you whisper.

Exactly! Every day should be filled with wonderful, ideal patients, but who are they? Where did they come from, and how can you get more?

When you're just getting started, anyone with a chiropractic problem who's willing to pay for your help looks ideal. However, as you've probably discovered by now, some patients cause more trouble than they're worth. It's not that we don't want them to get chiropractic; we just want them to get chiropractic someplace else.

To avoid this, smart DCs ask at least three questions:

- Who is my ideal patient?
- How do I get more just like them?
- How do I make it easy for them to find me?

If you get this wrong, the smile your morning coffee puts on your lips can be erased by the mere thought of going to the office. Who wants to spend their day arguing with negative complainers about following good-care recommendations, only to find out that they're also ninety days behind on their payments?

If you get this right, the most grateful people you know will thank you for doing what you love to do, and they'll refer their friends. That's when chiropractic is no longer work—it's your passion—turned hobby—turned incredible energy source. Goodbye, TGIF; hello, TGIMonday!

Let's start by identifying our ideal patient. This is a fun and productive exercise:

Think of seven patients you truly love caring for. We'll call them the Magnificent Seven. Ask your staff members to list their seven favorites as well. Remember, your staff helps attract and keep these gems, so involving them helps your CAs practice ownership.

Next, during an office meeting, discuss what the Magnificent Seven all have in common.

I'm willing to bet your ideal patient is grateful, courteous, keeps their appointments on time, gets better, pays their bill, refers their friends, and stays under care because they understand chiropractic. Hey, is perfect too much to ask?

Now it's a simple question of understanding what attitudes and procedures attract and teach what we want in a patient, while filtering out what we don't want in a patient.

#1: We want patients who are grateful and courteous.

Those attitudes start at the top. Do you express gratitude and courtesy to your staff? Your staff mirrors your attitude on to your patients, who reflect how they are treated back to the practice. Are you grateful for good work and courteous about requests?

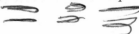

Hot tip: Give a sincere compliment to each staff person every day for a specific part of their job that's well done. If you do, your patients will be treated better—I promise.

#2: We want patients who are on time.

You guessed it—the way to get that is to be on time yourself. Nothing fouls a finely-tuned practice machine more often than a doctor who runs behind. Want to see twelve patients an hour? Don't keep running at eight to ten an hour.

Insist that patients have multiple-appointment plans, which can project order into your future.

For the person who wants to bring their own brand of personal chaos into your day by always being late, have your CA handle them like this: "Oh, Karen, I'm sorry you're late, too. I can't get you in right now, but Dr. Lloyd has an opening and can see you in forty-five minutes, after his regularly scheduled appointments. Do you want to get a latte and come back then?"

Please don't let Karen cut the line. By being firm about your policies, you're protecting your ideal patients and filtering out chaos. Remember, you're training patients, or your patients will be training you.

Hot tip: Ask your front desk to be direct with you on how you do with time.

#3: We want patients who get better.

Chiropractors with the highest certifications in their chosen techniques, who insist on complete care plans, get the best clinical results.

It's sad, but not everyone gets better under our care. However, let's not let that be due to sloppy work or our own failure to insist on strictly following a great care plan.

Hot tip: Pretend you'll receive a $10,000 bonus for the best care plan, laid out in advance and enforced to the end. What would that look like?

#4: We want patients who pay.

Even the best chiropractic care plans can create financial problems for most patients. Create humane patient payment plans to handle deductibles, copays and non-covered services. Then give your patients a choice of acceptable options to pay you.

"But, Noel, what if the patient can't afford any of the options?" This is where your policy becomes a filter to protect you. Instead of struggling with patients who can't pay, care for those who can and do.

"What about the patient who agrees to pay then defaults on their promise?" You need a system to act as another filter. Train your CA to say, "Oh, Karl, if I can't keep your account current, I can't extend credit. I'm going to need the payment we agreed on."

On one occasion, I listened to my CAs send a patient home to get the wallet he'd "forgotten" three times already, insisting he pay his bill before they'd let him in to get adjusted.

Hot tip: Most of the bad debt in your clinic is an attitude, policy, and enforcement problem.

#5: We want patients who refer their friends.

At the peak of their excitement about chiropractic, tell your ideal patient, "Janet, I'd love ten more patients just like you."

In my New Patient Orientation class, I say, "Tonight I'll teach you who needs to see a chiropractor and how to make a referral." Then I do what I promised and give them certificates for free consultations and exams to give to friends and family.

Hot tip: Make your top referring patient the patient of the month. Watch the interest and friendly competition grow among your ideal patients.

#6: We want patients who stay under care because they understand chiropractic and know it's in their best interest.

If we want them to "get it," we need to "give it" in a way they understand. I learned that the hard and expensive way.

Early in my own practice, I became disappointed with the number of maintenance patients I had. I hired a market research company to find out why for me. The short answer they uncovered was my patients loved me but didn't think they needed any more chiropractic.

What?

I was shocked. How could they have missed the message? Then I quit blaming them and decided that I would take responsibility to fix that. I sat down with each patient individually, as their care plan was ending, and explained maintenance and wellness again. I offered them a chance to sign up for a monthly adjustment.

In twenty-two months, I signed more than 480 patients into a simple monthly adjustment program. We started by loading as many as we could onto Tuesdays. On one Tuesday, we saw over eighty maintenance patients. It was truly an ideal day. The whole house was full of the best patients I knew.

Hot tip: Build a group of patients in your practice who make a full-year commitment to maintenance or wellness care. Start scheduling them all on Tuesdays, and watch Tuesday become your favorite day of the week.

#7: We want to make it easy for ideal patients to find us.

I don't think it's too simplistic to ask that we be the ideal doctor great patients are looking for.

That being said, I believe it's always on us to tell the chiropractic story and to be witnesses to the miracles we have been blessed to watch, literally at arm's length.

It's on us to take those stories out of the office in whatever way will bring the sick and suffering face-to-face with the opportunity to become patients who are grateful, courteous, keep their appointments, show up on time, get better, pay their bills, refer their friends, and stay under care because they understand chiropractic.

Hot tip: Don't give up.

4

What's the Real Problem Here? *TOO FEW NEW*

"I don't have enough new patients." This, in my opinion, is the single biggest problem facing the chiropractic profession. I could probably get a debate from someone, but they'd lose.

For more than twenty-five years, "too few new" has been the number one reason chiropractors have sought my advice and guidance, by a factor of twelve to one.

To further prove the point, when a doctor really gets the new patient problem handled, their professional life changes, big time and wonderfully. It's not that things become perfect—they're never perfect—but they get to deal with a classier set of problems, such as "Doctor, where do we put them all? When can we get an associate to help out? Doctor, we need more wall space for these patient testimonies. Doctor, we need a bigger office!" Or the popular/unpopular, "My quarterly tax payments are WHAT?"

I like those problems a lot more than wondering if someone has cut my phone lines or nailed my door shut. Or "Doctor, it's the bank. They're saying my paycheck won't clear again. What should I tell them?" Ouch.

It's simple: Get new patients right, and things are fun and exciting. Get new patients wrong, and you struggle miserably.

It's even more critical: You can get *everything else* right and new patients wrong, and you're in for a very rough, unpleasant ride. It's that important.

But don't feel singled out for punishment here. All businesses—and chiropractic is a business—depend on attracting new customers to survive. A lack of new customers is the reason most small businesses fail.

So why is it that so many of us resent the fact that our practices are businesses? And even more, why do we absolutely hate the fact that we have to market what we do to an uninformed (or misinformed) public?

"I've never seen an MD do a mall screening," I heard a colleague sneer.

I actually have, but that's beside the point. Ordinary medicine has the most sophisticated, well-financed marketing and advertising on the planet. Big Pharma—a $1.1 trillion worldwide industry—spends billions of dollars every year shilling, 24/7, for its distributors in every media possible. Try to watch TV, surf the Internet, read a magazine, or drive down the street and not be bombarded with drug advertisements. Oh, and by the way, if symptoms persist, see your doctor.

That is never going to happen for us in chiropractic, but that's okay. We are not victims, and it's dangerous to think like one.

When are we going to embrace that we're in business and that virtually all businesses need to market and advertise for new customers in order to flourish?

Jesus admonished the disciples to be wise as serpents and harmless as doves, and that's still good advice. But what is the wisdom we need here?

Thinking correctly about marketing—not jumping into the next desperate "Hail Mary" effort—is the first step. Over the past four decades in my own clinics and advising others, I've developed a set of postulates, which I share here with a promise: **Embrace these concepts, and you will produce more new patients.** Additionally, you'll have an excellent chance of beating the new patient problem.

Ready? Here we go:

1. Accept that it's not unethical to tell the truth about the benefits of chiropractic *outside your office,* and then give people a chance to find out if they can live better and longer lives with chiropractic. *Marketing honestly*

2. Because no one else will, you must do *all sorts* of external marketing to spread the truly good news we have to share. And by all sorts, I mean anything and everything that's legal, ethical, and produces new patients. *Why not? love the process*

3. Get over the "I am not a salesperson!" thing. Truth be told, everyone's a salesperson. Pastors, teachers, and coaches are selling to their congregations, students, and players. If you have an idea that you want someone to embrace, you're a salesperson. The only question is, are you any good at it?

4. Spend three to seven hours a week thinking and acting like the marketing director for yourself, chiropractic, and your practice. Choose what to do based on what works in your area and your personal taste.

5. Take your three to seven hours to develop a marketing Six-Pack—three internal and three external programs to produce new patients.

6. When your business can support it, train a part-time community outreach assistant (COA) to do everything you need to in

external marketing, leaving you in the clinic to care for your patients.

It's enough to bring tears to your eyes when you walk to the front desk and see your COA writing in between six and eight new appointments. "Doctor, we had a great event, with tons of new patient signups, and they've invited us back next month! Doctor, are you crying?" Yes, the doctor is crying, but they're tears of joy.

Even though I know an increasing number of chiropractors who have waiting-list practices based solely on referrals, most practices need to market to be as busy as they would like to be. Since that's the case, doesn't it make sense to have a staff person designated to marketing? But how many have a written job description for a marketing assistant?

When opening a new clinic—and I opened ten—my first hire was always a community outreach assistant. And because I'm good at developing this position, I did very well with attracting new patients.

Challenge: Do you want to love your busy practice? Do you want someone to go get the new patients for you while you stay in the clinic and care for patients? Then package all your external marketing into teachable systems and train your first COA. Don't stop until you become the Ninja Sensei of the COA!

5

Chiropractic Marketing 101

There's nothing—and I mean *nothing*—that will change your practice and your life like getting good at getting new patients. When new patient stats are up, so is your mood and the energy in the clinic. The practice is a wonderful place to be, and the day flies by. Services are up, collections are better, and bills get paid on time. Life's a ball.

When new patients are down, everything is a struggle, and nothing's any fun. For many practices, this is the way things are all the time. **The average chiropractor sees 4.3 new patients a week, sees fewer than one hundred visits a week, and struggles with attracting new patients throughout their entire time in practice.**

Yet it doesn't have to be that way.

With so many DCs struggling with new patients, why in the world doesn't every single one of us become a student of chiropractic marketing? Why don't we all do whatever's necessary to become experts at internal and external new patient chiropractic promotions?

The way many chiropractors market chiropractic, themselves, and their practice would be laughable if it weren't so painful to watch, and if there wasn't so much at stake.

Every year DCs put an offer for a free exam on the back of grocery store register tape, right next to the "$5 off your next large pizza" offer, hoping to get new patients. Why? Because they're desperate and don't know Chiropractic Marketing 101. I even know a DC who paid to place his free consultation and exam offer on the inside of restroom stall doors. I guess he wanted new patients to read all about chiropractic at their leisure.

I repeat: it doesn't have to be this way.

Why do nice, sane people make crazy decisions like that? They're grasping at straws because they don't know what else to do.

The awful truth is that it isn't enough to be a great, compassionate person who knows how to set an atlas perfectly or adjust a lumbar with great skill in order to succeed in practice.

I know wonderful chiropractors who now do other work because they never got the new patient thing right.

So I'm going to share with you a brief set of concepts, principles, and strategies that will allow you to pick the programs that really produce new patients. Use them effectively until they actually work, and you'll continue to produce new patients.

A full 90 percent of non-healthcare businesses would fail if they adopted the most common DC marketing strategies. That's because many DCs view marketing as a type of punishment for being a bad doctor. That's not true. There are always chiropractors who think marketing is beneath them. They say, "I don't do sales; I'm a doctor." *If you're passionate about an idea, you can sell it* Doctors, everyone is a salesperson.

Think of it this way: Parents are "selling" kids on getting good grades and keeping good company. Kids are "selling" parents on staying up later and needing a new cell phone. Pastors, coaches, and teachers are selling congregations, teams, and students. Anyone who has an idea that they want others to embrace is a salesperson. The only question is, are you any good at sales?

Get good at sales, and your practice will be great. Look down your nose at sales, and you'll struggle in practice. It's that simple.

You must do something.

Most DCs answer "none" when asked how many hours they spend each week on marketing outside their practice. Usually that's because they don't know what to do. However, successful practitioners of Chiropractic Marketing 101 know that they should spend three to seven hours weekly at internal and external marketing. These hours are scheduled in the appointment book and have specific activities or events associated with them.

They increase their skills over time and diversify their new patient programs through a Chiropractic Marketing Six-Pack, which we'll explore in a later chapter. They always do the tried and true, *and* they always try the brand new thing. They become a student of marketing principles and concepts.

Imagine the time you would put into a hobby that paid you an extra $250,000 a year.

They also embrace a new set of attitudes. They're never quitters, believing "if so-and-so can do it, so can I." They decide on the results they want, master the skills, and then pass on the skills to others.

I've seen hundreds of practices changed as a result of learning Chiropractic Marketing 101, including a woman who added 175 visits a week to her practice and trained a marketing assistant who still produces twelve to twenty new patients a week. Then there's the man who added 180 visits a week to his practice, and another woman who now has a six-to-eight-week waiting list for new patients in her practice.

So dust off what worked best in the past and commit to doing it again for two hours a week. Then let's look at new patient concepts, strategies, and programs!

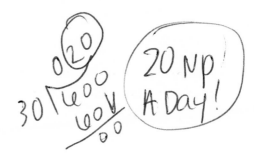

6

Imagine Seeing 601 New Patients in a Month

I enjoy opening workshops for chiropractors with that statement. It's designed to elicit a strong reaction, and I've gotten many—from cheers and laughter, to some shudders, to a few grimaces, to an occasional "No thank you!"

It took me a while to understand the negative responses. I discovered that some DCs picture how hard they work to acquire and process just a *few* new patients, and then they imagine that stretching their systems over such a big number could produce spontaneous combustion ("Hey, Doc just burst into flames in the X-ray room!").

My practice actually did produce 601 new patients in one thirty-one-day period. We later referred to that achievement just as "the 601." It was a wild and wooly month, to be sure.

However, it's the back story on the 601 that's interesting and instructive. A full 80 percent of those patients were from external marketing efforts, and I didn't do any of the outside work. I also didn't explode in the X-ray room. In fact, I had a lot of fun that month...and every month since.

Here's the setup:

Years before the 601, I'd learned how to do many variations of spinal screenings outside the office, at venues including festivals, fairs, malls, corporate (maxi and mini) health fairs, and club events. We did them all, and we did them well.

From the start, I made screening all about having fun. "Fun is Job One!" was my mantra. "Fun first; get new patients second." My attitude was if you're having fun, you attract more people and meet new patients.

But this chapter is about me *not* doing the outside work. How did I shift from super screener to super event manager?

I soon needed help at screenings for greeting, prepping, appointing, and following up on prospects, so I hired two community outreach assistants. At the same time, I was running an associate training center that was working extremely well. Some of my associates had grown to three hundred, four hundred, and even five hundred visits a week. If training worked that well for associates, I thought, I should run a short weekly training for new COAs. Before long, the COAs and I were all on the same page as to how to run events.

Immediately, my external marketing worked better and was less stressful. We role-played in COA training, and then I inspected and corrected at the events. I'd go back, update my notes, and upgrade my training systems. I was learning at least as much as the COAs.

A couple of eager young women who'd done well at COA training kept asking for more hours, so I started having them pick up the screening equipment, precede me to the event, set up, and even survey the group and make a list of people who wanted to get checked.

I'd arrive in time to screen people, have fun, make appointments, give departing instructions, and leave. The COAs stayed to pack up the gear, head back to the clinic, and put the new patients in the schedule.

"Hey, this is getting pretty easy," I thought.

One night, I sent my favorite COA to set up and wait for me. By the time I arrived, she'd already made three appointments. She'd taken it upon herself to learn my screening script. Some of you are thinking, "I'd never go to a screening myself again! I'd send her!" However, that isn't the way I handled it—at least not then.

On another screening night, I was detained at the clinic for an emergency new patient. I got to the event about the time it was supposed to end and found my COA had booked six new patients. She asked to try an event solo. Permission granted!

After that, I added equal parts opportunity and responsibility. That COA became a co-trainer for other COAs. Eventually she developed sites, ran her own events, and headed up teams.

Now, are you ready for the story of the 601? Along with my associates, I had seventeen full- and part-time COAs who, all combined, produced the 601 for eight doctors in five clinics. One clinic saw more than 150 new patients that month —all of it administrated by two COAs.

I never worked one event during that 601 month.

Here are the three keys that have served me very well ever since:

1. I find genetically gifted COA applicants and screen out the duds.

2. Properly trained, nearly all COAs can produce new patients without me in less than a month.

3. With daily—yes, *daily* (this is key)—guidance, motivation, and correction, COAs can produce an extra five or more new

patients a week, and keep producing for months, even years. The average is 4.2 new patients a week, without the doctor having to be at the event.

I've hired many COAs over my forty years in practice. Some have been exceptional, and some didn't last a week, but even the average COAs produced many times what they cost.

7

Five Modern Strategies to Expand Your Patient Base

This chapter title needs a little clarification. What do I mean by "modern"?

The best marketing strategy produces the most qualified new patients, even if that strategy has been around for decades. Additionally, just because something is new and comes in a glitzy package with slick promises doesn't mean it works. The modern strategies you want will be a combination of the brand new and the tried and true, where everything works seamlessly.

Modern Strategy #1: Diversify.

Investment counselors tell us we should keep our portfolio varied, and I agree. In chiropractic marketing, I call it a "Six-Pack" of new patient programs—three internal and three external, with all six independent programs functioning simultaneously.

If you diversify, you'll always have new patients from several sources. Those who diversify their marketing always have at least one or two programs they can move forward, even when another one or two are stuck. And if your experience is like mine, there'll be a top-dog program in each set of three, with a second and then the runt of the litter. We're always looking for a new thing to beat the weakest internal and external programs.

Internal Marketing Example: Every office should have a program for complimentary consults and exams. Give a well-designed complimentary visit certificate to excited patients to help them refer friends or family.

I also love eliciting, collecting, and displaying patient testimonies. We have a testimony form that we use as an outline when the DC or CA have time to do an interview or that we can send home with the patient if we're too busy. We keep all the testimonies in three books in our offices and frame the best for the walls.

Hot tip: Every new patient I've met in the past sixty years heard a positive chiropractic story before they made an appointment, so keep the topic of new testimonies in your office meeting agenda as a reminder to keep the supply fresh. Video testimonies are great for your website, but paper is best in the office.

External Marketing Example: I love corporate events like health fairs and massage days. They will put your practice in front of employed people with good insurance who work close by— good prospects. Tell your current patients you're putting together your public service calendar for the next few months, and ask them to check their company calendars to see if there's something appropriate for you.

Hot tip: Have a public service bulletin board in your office with pictures of your team serving at corporate events, along with the follow-up thank you letters on company letterhead. You'll start to hear, "Doctor, I'm organizing our health fair this year, and I saw those pictures. Would you come to our health fair?"

Modern Strategy #2: Show your calendar you're serious about marketing.

For most of us, our calendar is our appointment book. So *schedule* three to seven hours of real time every week to work on marketing.

If what you're committed to never shows up on your schedule, you're not committed—just a big talker.

Initially, it may take seven hours a week to produce just three extra new patients. When you get really good at your Six-Pack, you can reverse those numbers and produce seven (or more) extra new patients a week with just three hours.

Hot Tip: Create more marketing time in your calendar by close scheduling your early morning and afternoon appointments, clearing the middle of the day. You'd be surprised how many corporate events are scheduled between 10:00 and 2:00.

Modern Strategy #3: Apply the Rule of Fives.

If you want to be slim, forget the latest diet book. Just ask five slim people what and how much they eat. Then do the same. If you want to be fit, find five fit people, and work out like they do. I promise you this strategy is 100 percent successful.

I was at a seminar where a fit guy who seemed to be my age was working a booth. I approached him and asked what his health and fitness routine was. Guess what: he doesn't drink much, gets his carbs from vegetables and fruit, and keeps the workout weights light and reps heavy because "it saves on the joints, and you'll never dread your workout." Good advice that works.

What do the top five chiropractic marketers do to get more clients? You may not like everything they do, or the way they do it, but it's a very modern doctor who finds out what the successful practices are doing and does the same thing. Before you know it, you're one of the five.

Hot Tip: You can share the cost of some bigger events with your group of five. For example, my practice split the cost and time commitment of marketing at a seventeen-day state fair with others in our area.

Modern Strategy #4: "It's not my strategy—it's my commitment to my strategy."

The first time I heard that sentence it sank deep into my soul. Seldom do you hear that much truth in so few words.

Instead of desperately flinging a half-backed marketing concept at the wall to see if it sticks, take the time to study, plan, and commit to making your plan work. Old fashioned? Of course, but it's the only way to beat the new patient problem in a modern world. *need) to true*

The first time I did a screening, I headed up a team of eight doctors who checked well over five hundred people, yet we didn't make one appointment. I simply didn't know how. Years later, we welcomed more than six hundred new patients in one month into my clinics —mainly from screenings. I was committed to my strategy and did not give up.

Hot Tip: Decide now that you'll become the expert in your area in at least one marketing program and never give up.

Marketing Strategy #5: Develop marketing assistants to do your marketing.

This is my favorite modern strategy. DCs have CAs who help us route and process patients, right? So why don't we all have community outreach assistants (COAs) to help us bring in large numbers of qualified new patients?

Learn to package what you're doing that's working and teach it to an assistant so they can continue to produce new patients while you stay in the clinic and dream up other marketing programs to keep your clinic full.

I've gotten much better at finding someone who is genetically gifted at sales, training them correctly, and then managing the position, but the bottom-line strategy is always the same: Take the skills that I've acquired and train a COA.

Hot Tip: Creating training templates for tools is a breeze. New patient programs with simple tools (SAM machines, clipboards, screening forms, free exam certificates) are easy to design and replicate if you create a script and proper use for each tool.

Imagine you've taken a patient to the front desk for some reason, and you run into your marketing assistant, who's just back from an event. She greets you with a smile and mouths the number twelve. "Doctor, we met so many nice people at our outreach event today." She discreetly waves twelve new patient sign-up sheets at you. Now that's a modern success story.

8

The Five Things That Keep Patients from Coming to Your Office

People have been calling me for close to thirty years, asking me to help them correct or not make the common mistakes that keep patients from ever coming into their offices. And every year I consider what I've heard and make an intense study of the current top five mistakes great chiropractors make that keep them from seeing enough new patients—and consequently fail at building the practices they've always dreamed they would.

Mistake #1: A poorly produced website that keeps people away in droves

Your website is the first place most prospective new patients see you—and that includes most referrals. "Jim liked this guy. I think I'll Google him."

I don't know what your website looks like, but when I was critiquing a client's site the other day, I was amazed to see there wasn't a large, simple button that said "New Patients HERE," or "Start HERE." There wasn't even a phone number on the home page!

I struggled through the nearly impossible-to-read copy looking for that phone number. I finally found it on an obscure subpage, in a font so hard to decipher I had to squint to read it. I'm convinced this website hurt more than it helped.

My critique and suggestions for him—and for you—are simple, direct, and work. Here they are:

- Make the instructions about how to make a new patient appointment and get into the office super-simple and easy to understand.
- Include pictures of doctors and staff in friendly individual and staff team photos.
- Add a two-minute "welcome to our office" video tour led by the doctor. This is easy to do with just the camera on your smart phone.

By the time people are on your site, they already know they want a chiropractor. A long, detailed explanation on how chiropractic works might actually hurt your web efforts by getting in the way and confusing people.

Hot Tip: Remember, less is more—as long as there's a big button in the upper right corner that promises a visitor that they can "Get Started NOW!"

Mistake #2: Not having new-patient friendly phone procedure

People learn how to find you on the web, but they make their first appointment by phone.

When I call some businesses, I wonder how they stay in business. The line rings too many times, and then I'm put on hold without my permission, and when they get back to me, I get the sense they just aren't ready for me or my business.

Here's my shortlist for avoiding phone mistakes:

- Always answer by the third ring.
- Practice a short, standard, and cheerful greeting: "Our Chiropractic Center, Mandy speaking. I can help you."
- Follow with courteous phone etiquette that promises you won't lose them. "In case we're disconnected, Jason, is (repeat caller ID#) the best number to reach you?"
- Create a "right now" policy with your staff. Once you know it's a new patient, don't put them off until tomorrow. They'll call the next office on their Google search. Part of your phone procedure needs to be "Is there any reason you can't come over right now?"

Hot Tip: Have the phones forwarded to an office cell number after hours, and give a motivated and trained CA a bonus for each new patient they book in the evenings and weekends. You'll be amazed how many new patient calls you're missing now.

Mistake #3: A shabby, rundown look that says you don't care

As a consultant, I request that all of my new clients send me a photo or video tour of their offices, starting from across the street or parking lot, taking me though the front door into reception and then through the entire office. I review, critique, and offer suggestions to make your office look more inviting to walk-by or drive-by prospects.

Sometimes what I see scares me.

To start with, clean up the parking lot, sidewalks, flower beds, blinds, and windows. Freshen up with a brand-new welcome mat, a new accent color for your door, or vinyl window graphics with your logo. And kill the clutter in reception.

Hot Tip: Have your spouse or a friend with a discerning eye give you a critique, and make suggested changes that you can tackle immediately. Momentum is important.

Mistake #4: Not having customer-service-centered new patient procedures

Years ago, I was greeted at a luxury hotel by a VIP concierge who made me feel like royalty. The woman stepped from behind the desk to greet me with a warm handshake. "Dr. Lloyd, my name is Teresa. How very nice to meet you." She wanted to know how my flight was, did I want sparkling or still spring water, and may she invite me into the VIP registration suite?

It was well done, and as far as I could tell, not that expensive—just polished and practiced courtesy.

I was so impressed that I wrote up a new procedure for greeting patients in my offices. It starts with the first phone call, becomes more personal as they enter the office, and extends to meeting the doctor. Our goal is a warm, personal experience that shows we care about the patient.

I love hearing my front desk CA say, "You must be Kate. My name is Mandy. It's nice to meet you and welcome to Sound Chiropractic."

Hot Tip: Script a greeting, with a helpful explanation of your initial paperwork, and then practice it with your staff until it's the way you want it.

Mistake #5: Not doing external marketing

After decades of study, I know that the best way to build a strong practice quickly is through external marketing. Not letting people know who you are and what you do is the same as hiding your practice from thousands of people in your community.

Ordinary medicine has a pharmaceutical industry worth several hundred billion dollars that is constantly schilling for it, telling people in every media possible that "if symptoms persist, see your doctor."

But we don't have that, so if chiropractors don't take the very attractive chiropractic message to their community, who will?

I conducted a patient focus group for one of my offices. We invited seven of our best patients to be our lunch guests, with the understanding that I'd ask them questions about what they liked or didn't like about our clinic.

"How did you hear about us?" I asked the group. A gracious woman with silver hair answered first. "I met the doctor at the mall. I was so impressed that he'd take his time to help people that way. I did that posture thing, and I was really a mess back then."

This wonderful lady had been a faithful wellness patient for years. But I wasn't prepared for what followed. Six of my seven guests—all our most cherished patients—also came to hear about us because of external marketing. And they all thought we stood above other offices because of what another patient called our "chiropractic missionary" work.

Hot Tip: In a way that suits your personality, package the chiropractic message, and take it to a world that desperately needs it. I promise you'll meet the best people in your community, and they'll be grateful you took the time.

Here's another promise: all these fixes are easy to do and inexpensive and will help you care for more people, have more fun, and be more successful.

9

The Chiropractic Marketing Six-Pack

Every DC has to be smart about marketing. For someone who knows they need to get more new patients and are willing to market, here's my strategy:

Make it official. Start your own "Double Your New Patients Project," and set aside three to seven hours of your time each week—not the scant twenty or thirty minutes here or there.

I've polled scores of doctors who say they need new patients, but when I ask how many hours they currently spend per week making a presentation, doing a demonstration, or extending an invitation outside the office, the most common answer is a big goose egg.

After you make the commitment of three to seven hours, diversify your efforts into three internal and three external programs— what I call the "Chiropractic Marketing Six-Pack."

Start with what you know to do, but which has fallen into disrepair. Then move on to something you always thought you'd be good at but haven't acted on.

Here are three no-cost examples of internal marketing programs:

Example #1: Set a new patient goal with your staff. Don't make it so high that it won't happen, but shoot for five visits above your average. Offer bonuses of $50-$100 per staff person if you all as a team reach the goal. Then brainstorm together which patients have talked about their friends or family, and make a note to have a conversation with those patients to offer a free consultation certificate for their friend or family member.

Example #2: Two to three times a day, bring patients with great chiropractic recovery stories up to the front desk and say, "Judy, please tell Mandy what you just told me in the adjusting area." When Judy tells her story—validating chiropractic and the work of the office—you'll feel the energy go up while the goals of your practice become more meaningful.

Coincidentally, you're also teaching patients that telling others about their experience is good.

Example #3: Have each staff person call two inactive patients a day with a simple and light touch reactivation script: "Judy, Dr. Lloyd asked me to give you a call. He's worried about you and wants you to schedule for a checkup. What day this week or next works best?"

As for external marketing, an Internet presence is a must. But spending big money on online gimmicks you don't understand is a big mistake. If you need help, real, valuable Internet coaching is affordable and pay-as-you-go. Ask any consultant you interview for a couple of references of similar businesses, and then call them.

Outside the office, screenings, lectures, and health fairs produce the best results and are the least expensive.

Here's a great project that's inexpensive and can hit pure gold: Put a CA on the phone with list of local companies to offer your practice's help with their upcoming health fairs. Offer free SAM screenings at a two- or three-hour midday event, and make appointments for follow-up office visits. I have clients who do one or two company health fairs a month, for an extra eight to ten new patients a month.

If you're nervous about change, do the cheaper, easier things that are similar to what you've done in the past first, then ramp up to bigger projects.

10

How to Use Spinal Screenings to Attract New Patients

Spinal screenings have proven to be a marketing strategy that produce a high number of new patients at a relatively low cost for most chiropractic practices. In addition to generating new patients, the people who you meet during screenings help develop your personal network.

The more people you know and the more activities you're involved with, the better off you will be.

Remember what happens to the people we don't meet: more drugs, more surgery, and other silly medical methods to address conditions that chiropractic alone is best suited to address.

There are many different types of setups for screenings. Generally speaking, the more people you screen, the more new patient invitations you give out. The more invitations you give out, the higher the number of people who will come to your office. And the more people who come to your office, the more new patients will begin chiropractic care.

My goal when screening is to generate at least one new patient per screening hour. But this is just the base; I have seen hundreds of screenings that generate more than ten new patients per hour.

The following are steps to guide you through the actual screenings, once you have a time and place scheduled.

Step 1: Setup

Whether you are setting up a small, medium, or large screening, look as professional as possible. Make sure that you are as visible as possible. If you are using signage, it should be fresh and clean. All paperwork should be first generation, clean copies.

The doctor's attire should be professional—a dress-casual shirt or a shirt and tie, or the equivalent for women—depending on the site. Assistants should be in uniform; golf shirts and khakis work well in most cases.

After arriving on site, set up and prepare to screen. I prefer the following equipment for a medium setup: a SAM or Myovision (or other) screening device, signage, two folding chairs, a plastic spine, between three and five clipboards, and all necessary paperwork. I set the two chairs up face-to-face, with the spine next to them. I use this area to talk to the prospects and then walk them to and from the SAM or Myovision device.

Step 2: Attraction

While you are doing a screening, your job is to interact with the public. Whether you're at a mall or visiting a private company, try to communicate with each person that you come in contact with.

Ask people:

- Would you like to get your spine checked? It takes two minutes, and it's totally painless.

- Would you like to have an ergonomic posture check?
- *What's wrong?* (to the person who's obviously in bad shape)

If the above questions aren't working, or if you want to change the pace, you can also try to engage people in other conversation: the weather, sports, or news of the day (but try to avoid religion, politics, or sex).

If you are not screening at least three people per hour, you probably should not be at the event, or else you really need to open your mouth more. I know many doctors who are uncomfortable promoting themselves. While you should work to have others promote you whenever possible, if you can't promote yourself, then your progress will be significantly slowed.

Step 3: Consultation

After a person agrees to be checked, I have them fill out a screening form. I get their address, phone number, and insurance information, as well as what clinically is bothering them. I then ask them about any of the symptoms they checked off. I will go through the PQRST pain assessment and other questions until one of two realities becomes clear: either the person has a health problem that they're concerned about or they don't.

If I am not sure, I will ask, "If you could leave all of the problems with your pain behind, would you want to?" If they answer yes or have already indicated that they are concerned about their health, I proceed on to a thorough screening. If they don't qualify, I screen them quickly and give them advice to get a full chiropractic exam if appropriate.

By the end of the consultation, I know if they qualify, and I also know:

- Where they work and live
- If they have a problem that they want help with

- If they have some way to pay (insurance, accident coverage, or a last name like Kennedy)

Step 4: The Screening

Regardless of how you are screening (SAM, EMG, Posture Pro, blood pressure, Metrecom, or other device), the goal is to have the person understand how a positive screening finding (high shoulder, weight differential, red or nonbilateral EMG readings, abnormal blood pressure, poor posture) is related to their spine. This damage to the structure or function of their spine can pinch, choke off, or irritate the nerve, which can be the cause of their problem.

During the screening, I will perform the test and then explain it to the person, trying to create as many of these connections (I call them *physical ahas*) as possible.

For example, if I am using a SAM, I set the strings at the level of the person's ears, shoulders, and hips, as well as view their lateral posture. Then I will explain my findings like this:

"Mary, if you look at these strings, they represent the level of your ears, shoulders, and hips. Do you see the problem? Your head is tilted to the right, your left shoulder is higher than the right, and the right hip is higher than the left. You also carry your head significantly forward over your body. Lastly, your weight differential is twelve pounds more on the right."

If the prospect is there with anyone else, like a spouse, sibling, or friend, I will have the other person confirm my findings. If I am in a really good mood, I might have the other person do the screening. I will also answer any questions right there at the SAM.

Step 5: Transition to Close

At this point, I take the person back to the chairs, and I grab the spine. I show them that if their spine is out of place, their nerves can be pinched. I may stick their pinky into a lumbar IVF and pinch it to demonstrate. I go on to explain that when this occurs, it may cause symptoms like theirs.

Step 6: The Close

I will then use my "million-dollar close." Over decades of practice and conversations with hundreds of doctors, I have found that using this close on qualified prospects (they have a problem they want help with, are close enough to get to your office, and have a way to pay) will close at least half.

"Mary, from the look of your screening, you may have some serious structural damage in your spine. If it were me, I would get it examined, and examined thoroughly. In my office when we examine people, we do over sixty tests to check muscles, bones, and nerves. The exam is designed to tell me two things. First, what is really causing the problem. And second, whether or not chiropractic would help it. Normally this exam is $65 (or whatever your fee is), but in conjunction with this event, I've set aside a small number of appointments to provide the exam at no charge. There are two conditions to the offer. The first is that you're serious about finding out more about your health, and the second is that you schedule the appointment today for later this week or next week. Don't take one if you aren't going to use it, but if I offered you a free exam, would you use it?"

Note: You may have a different offer than a free exam. I have seen $25 first visits (exam and X-rays) work well. I have also seen DCs take a $20 deposit that is returned when the patient shows up for the appointment.

If the person says yes, immediately schedule an appointment, giving them choices to keep them engaged and moving forward:

"What day is better for you, Monday or Tuesday? Morning or afternoon? 2:30 or 5:00?

"Carol, from our office, will call to make sure you know how to find us and to get some additional information for your file. What number is best?

"Great. The office is on Main Street, across from the police station. We'll see you on Tuesday at 5:00.

"Oh, one last thing, Mary. Missed appointments really affect us negatively in two ways. Is this something we need to talk about?"

This is known as a post-sale.

If they hedge at all, I will continue:

"I set aside this time for you, and I will meet with you personally. If there is any chance you won't be able to make this appointment, I would like to reschedule it now. By missing the appointment, you won't only not learn how chiropractic can help you, but someone else who would use the appointment slot won't be able to."

Step 7: Post Screening

When the screening is over, pack up, leave, and if possible, go back to the office. Put all the equipment away, and record your appointments immediately in your appointment book, spreadsheet, software, contact management, or however you keep your schedule and patients in one central location.

Step 8: Pre-Call

One to three days before the appointment, I start to pre-call my prospects. CAs can do this, but so can DCs. The script is as follows:

"This is Carol from Dr. Lloyd's office. The doctor told me that you met over the weekend and that you decided to take advantage of one of our Invitation to Health appointments. Did he also tell you that this is a no-charge visit designed to see if chiropractic can help you? I have your last name as Jones, J-O-N-E-S. Is that correct? Our office is located at 1927 Carson Street on the south side of the street. Where will you be coming from? (Make sure that your directions are specific.) The doctor usually runs on time, so if you could show up ten minutes early to fill out some paperwork, the doctor will see you right at your appointment time. Great, I look forward to meeting you tomorrow."

Step 9: Follow-Up

I call any missed new patient appointments until they come in, or until they tell me they're not interested anymore. If I can't reach them after two weeks, I add them to a mailing list that is contacted twice a year.

I try to have at least eight hours of screenings a month, with the goal of producing eight new patients. If you are not getting those results, try reviewing all of these steps, and make a list of things that could be improved.

The screening process can be blocked at any of the steps, so it's important to identify where you are stuck if things aren't working. Debugging is not only important but essential.

11

The Power of a Good Story

I was setting up for a screening when a man stopped and said, "A chiropractor saved my life."

He had seen the plastic spine, assumed I was a chiropractor, and wanted to tell his story. So I listened. It was an inspiring tale that gave me goose bumps, and after he'd finished, I shook his hand and thanked him for telling it to me. Seconds later, another man and his wife in a nearby booth said, "A chiropractor saved the life of my son's friend." They'd heard the first man's story and wanted to tell me *their* heart-warming story. I thanked them as well. I remember thinking, "Thank you, God, for letting me be a chiropractor." I felt great all day.

What lifts your spirits and energizes you, Doctor? What encourages and excites a CA about their job? What inspires people to tell their friends about chiropractic, and what moves people to pick up the phone and call to make a new patient appointment?

Patient testimonies—true-life stories of how extraordinary chiropractic is and how ordinary chiropractors change people's lives every day.

While most chiropractic practices collect patient testimonies, most doctors don't know how to fully utilize them. So let me show you how to artfully and consistently get and use patient testimonies to increase your practice enjoyment, energy, retention, *and* new patient referrals.

Getting the Story

A good chiropractic testimony is a three-part story including a *before*, an *encounter*, and an *after*. The *before* is a list of the bad things that made your patient miserable. The *encounter* is a brief story of how the patient met you and what starting care was like. The *after* is how the patient's life has changed for the better.

You'll need to prepare for this. Remind every staff member to always have time to listen to and be excited about every patient testimony. Also, keep testimony questionnaires in key areas of the office. The form is designed to extract the facts from the *before*, the *encounter*, and the *after* chiropractic.

Every week in your staff meeting, discuss patients' responses to care. SAs a team; select several patients to ask for testimonies. Mark their treatment card somehow with a note to follow up.

When the patient comes in, begin by saying, "Don, I know you're really progressing. Tell me how your life is better because of chiropractic." Stop and listen. What you'll hear will encourage you, so don't be afraid to let the patient know it does. "Don, I've been a chiropractor for almost forty years, and I never tire of hearing about how it helps people."

If you can, take the patient to reception and say to your front desk CA, "Don was just telling me how his care is coming along, and I thought you'd like to hear too." The CAs love seeing their patients' confidence in chiropractic get boosted. They know it's their job to listen and share their excitement. You're also teaching patients that they should share their chiropractic successes, and that both doctor and staff really care.

Plus, new and established patients may be listening in and be encouraged as well.

When they're finished sharing their story, either you or your CA should pull out a testimony questionnaire and say, "Don, we would be honored if you would share your story with our patients. Hearing chiropractic stories like yours is how most people get motivated to get the help they need. Sharing your story helps everyone." Most people are glad to share their success.

If the patient has time, ask them to fill out the form right there. Or use the form to interview the patient, looking for the most moving or emotional aspects of their story.

Take a digital picture of the patient to make the story more personal, and attach an intriguing headline. When chiropractic saved the patient from an operation, the title was: Dr. Lloyd Saves Woman from Knife Attack! Another title was: I Would Have Cut Off My Head and Given It to You! These titles make you want to read these stories.

Print and ask the patient to read, verify, and sign their testimony.

How to Use Testimonies

Here are just a few ways to use these testimonies in your office:

1. Make up three testimony books—two for your reception area and one to take to screenings. When I'm at a spinal screening and meet a migraine case, I show the individual the migraine testimonies.
2. Put each testimony in an inexpensive frame, and add it to your "glory wall." Highlight a new testimony by making them the "patient of the month," and teach your other patients to read the latest testimonies.

3. At each New Patient Orientation class, if you offer those, open the class by sharing one testimony, as well as your own personal perspective on that patient's search for help. You will give yourself more confidence and prepare the group for the chiropractic message.

4. Don't stop there. If your local laws permit, use testimonies in advertising and on your website.

Set a goal right now to collect fifty new testimonies in the next twelve months. It will change your practice for good.

12

Why Some Patients Vanish

"What happened to my 3:30 report of findings?"

Have you ever had to ask that? They may have rescheduled, but there are two all-too-common answers no chiropractor wants to hear:

"She called to cancel. I tried to get her to reschedule; she refused."

"She's a no-show. I called and left a message but haven't heard back."

With the number one challenge for most chiropractors being not having enough new patients, when someone comes in for Day One and then disappears, it's discouraging. I've been working on patient retention in general, and the one-visit problem specifically, for over forty years. What went so wrong on their first visit that they didn't want to hear what you found, see their X-rays, or start getting better?

"What did I do wrong?"

What indeed?

I heard a young pastor once explain that he was grateful for his critics, because of what they taught him. We can all learn from that. Can we put aside the excuses, irritation, or even hurt feelings that come from a no-show and be smart enough to learn from the never-to-return?

Experience tells me to first check three areas for problems:

1. What the patient sees: the office, staff, and doctor
2. How the patient is treated: the customer service
3. How the patient is cared for: the patient care

Visuals

You want to inspire confidence in your patients. However, there's no need to be palatial, just neat, clean, and fresh. Show them that you care about your look.

Here's my short list for a visual review:

1. Is there trash in the parking lot? An overflowing ashtray somewhere near your entrance? Even though you may not own the parking lot, it's "your" parking lot. Assign one of the CAs to outside trash detail, and inspect the space regularly.
2. Have someone with a discerning eye visit your office and give it the once-over. Take suggested upgrades seriously. When I had an active practice, every Tuesday I inspected my offices with the CAs tasked to keep things ship-shape and gave them a to-do list.
3. Dress the part. I won't preach here, but there are many studies showing patients prefer a uniformed staff and a doctor—clean shaven if you're male—wearing business attire.

Hot Tip: Ask one of your colleagues or Business Network International (BNI) buddies to trade critiques.

Customer Service

Many chiropractic offices grew up mimicking the bad influence of the ordinary doctor's practice, where "customer service" included a rude receptionist and a forty-five-minute wait in reception, followed by another thirty minutes of freezing in your underwear in the exam room before you see the doctor. Those were bad manners all around.

By contrast, great hotels and fine restaurants have customer care down to an art.

A few years ago, I made reservations at one of the country's best restaurants. When I arrived, I was treated like a king. "Dr. Lloyd, welcome to the Herb Farm. This must be your son. Chris, are you excited to head off to Wheaton?"

When I'd made the reservation, the receptionist asked if we were celebrating a special occasion. I said yes, my son had been accepted to Wheaton College. Over the course of the evening, no fewer than four staff congratulated Chris on his acceptance to his college of choice. We felt very special. Magic? No, just great training.

Now imagine you're a new chiropractic patient on Day One and not feeling well. Your coworker has already tried to talk you out of seeing a chiropractor, and you're walking into a strange office where you know no one.

You push open the sparkling-clean glass door and enter a neat reception area that's filled with pleasant music. The young woman behind the desk makes eye contact with a smile, stands, and walks around the counter to shake your hand. "You must be [your name here]. My name is Mandy. Welcome to Sound Chiropractic."

It's an impressive way to begin, and you're in a good place to hear the explanation of your intake forms.

How did she know who you were? Well, it's 2:15, and the front desk CA sees a new patient appointment in that slot. A stranger matching the right gender just walked in, so it was a good bet. It's not rocket science, just thoughtful customer service. And it tells the patient they're in the right place.

Hot Tip: Script and practice your CA's greeting to show your patient they're in an office that truly cares, and award a bonus to your CA each time you hear the script done right.

Now it's your turn: Hands down, the best way to ensure your patient comes back tomorrow is to do an excellent job connecting with them. Coming across as a caring expert on this first visit is even more important than the care itself.

For decades, I started my consultation with the following script. By the time I finished this sixty-second explanation, the patient and I were on the same page.

"Before we get started, I want to tell you how we do things here. I only have two concerns: what's wrong and can chiropractic help you. I'm a stickler for detail, and I'll ask a lot of questions. What I'm looking for are good, concise answers.

"When we're done talking, if I think I can help you, I'll tell you. If not, I'll try to find someone who can.

"I'm also concerned about cost containment and won't recommend any tests, X-rays, or treatment that aren't absolutely necessary.

"Finally, I believe in teamwork between doctor and patient. I think it's the reason I get the good results that I do. I ask my patients to work with me like a team. And if I accept your case, I'm going to ask you to work as hard as I do. Can I count on you for that? Great, now tell me all about..."

When I'm finished, I've told the patient I care, framed our roles, and asked for a commitment. The right patient is thrilled when you take control for their good.

My consulting clients—other chiropractors—tell me that this is the most powerful script they've ever used, too, and that it cuts in half their "one and done" problem of clients who never return.

Patient Care

This may sound counterintuitive, but I promise it's true: Doctors who feel compelled to do everything, including an adjustment, on the first visit have a much higher "one and done" rate and a lower patient visit average than those who take the time to properly analyze their exam and X-ray findings and bring the patient back the following day for their first adjustment.

As you release your patient on Day One, tell them that you'll analyze everything tonight and will review it all with them tomorrow.

In addition, make yourself strict about giving home-care instructions. Patients respect this. Then walk them up to the front desk, and explain to the CA what you both agreed on. By this point, when you tell them you'll see them tomorrow, you almost always do.

13

Creating Your "Wow" Experience

A few years ago, I scheduled Five Star Management's annual Galaxy meeting at the Ritz-Carlton hotel in Cancun, Mexico. Galaxy is the name of our mastermind group for high achievers. We choose interesting locations around the world and meet to share, challenge, and encourage each other in beautiful settings. Somehow I knew that everyone would be looking for a little tropical sunshine in mid-February.

We had booked the event solid and had worked out all the usual adjustments with the hotel to make sure the event was just right for our clients and for Five Star. The hotel was gracious and accommodating at every turn.

When I arrived a day before our guests, I was greeted by Sarah Peña from the Ritz-Carlton, and that's when the magic really began. I'll fast forward this for you and just say that everything the hotel touched was perfection. Each aspect of our stay was an example of what a first-class hotel can do to make their guests happy. I was thrilled, and so were my clients.

However, it was what happened just before I *left* the hotel that was not only impressive but instructive as well. It truly was a "wow" moment.

Let's go back to the first day I arrived. Sarah mentioned that before I left, she would like to have a post-event interview to see how the hotel and staff performed. I didn't think very much of it at the time, but the day before we concluded our meeting Sarah mentioned it again, and the morning of my departure, I received a reminder call about the meeting. I was starting to believe this was a very important conversation for this company. It was, and I learned a ton too.

Sarah's coworker, Antonio, met me in the lobby, where we sat in comfortable chairs as he asked me question after question about the hotel facilities, the staff, and my clients' comments about their stay. He asked for me to rate everything on a one-to-five scale.

The reason everything was perfect is because the Ritz-Carlton takes detailed notes like this on everything their experienced consumers say and then uses their findings to reward their star performers and improve everyone's performance.

So how can you take that to your own business? On Day One for new patients in your office, ask them to fill out a short comment card with the following questions:

1. Were you treated well on the phone when you called for your appointment?
2. Was it easy to get an appointment that worked for your schedule?
3. Were you greeted warmly and by name when you entered the office?
4. Did you see the doctor in a timely manner?

5. Were your health concerns addressed?

Now collect these cards, and review them with your staff, adjusting your checklists and training to produce the same five-star, exceptional service that the Ritz-Carlton trains for and delivers. Make a checklist of what you want your practice to deliver as exceptional customer service.

When a patient comes for a reevaluation or reexamination, you have another opportunity to ask them about their experience. Before their reexam, you or a CA can ask the following questions:

1. Is our staff courteous, and do they treat you well?
2. Do you have a good relationship with your doctor?
3. Are we educating and informing you about your health and chiropractic?
4. How do you feel about your care schedule?
5. Is your account being handled the way you like?
6. Are the clinic hours convenient?
7. Are you satisfied with your results?
8. Do you have any suggestions that you feel will help us take better care of you?

I've used this list of questions in my offices and my clients' offices for years. However, some clinic owners have told me that they weren't so sure they wanted to know the answers.

Here's an interesting statistic: 67 percent of customers or patients leave a service not because the service didn't work for them, but because of *how it was delivered*. In short, poor customer service is the major reason you lose good patients. That, if nothing else, should motivate you to ask the hard questions.

Patients are thinking about their experiences whether you ask or not. So why not find out if you're hitting the mark or falling short? You can use the responses to train staff as well. And your patients will be impressed that you care enough to find out.

14

Making the Visit Count

If I have any regrets surrounding chiropractic, it is that too many of my patients didn't follow through on good chiropractic care plans to get the "big picture" and the best that chiropractic has to give. I'm a lifetime chiropractic patient, so why aren't they?

The simple fact that so many patients just don't stick around long enough—poor patient compliance—became a serious study of mine. After spending thousands of dollars on research, over two years my practice went from a thirty-six PVA to a seventy-two PVA by applying a number of small but important fixes.

1. Do a head, heart, and gut check.

Are you giving "Golden Rule" recommendations?

Think about what care recommendations you would outline for your father, mother, sister, brother, spouse, or children. Are you offering the same to your patient? Remember, it's your responsibility to assess the patient's needs and make recommendations for the best care plan, not the cheapest or easiest.

When you give Golden Rule recommendations, you align your head, heart, and gut. Your conviction, compassion, and confidence increase. Additionally, if the road gets rough along the way, you know that you didn't hold anything back and can defend it.

Exercise: Based on your primary technique protocols, as well as your clinical experience, lay out a "Golden Rule" care plan for a hypothetical patient. Present the plan to a colleague, asking them to take the "devil's advocate" position and question your reasoning. Respond to each question with a smile and the starting phrase "Great question. Let me clarify..."

Special note: Let's assume that you don't adjust on the first day, and you instead schedule a Day Two report of findings. The next two tips must be part of a good ROF.

2. Have written care plans.

To help counteract the temptation to cut corners or hold back, prepare a written care plan designed to take each patient through relief, correction, and strengthening and into wellness. Written care plans make it harder to chicken out when recommending care.

Exercise: Write out your care plans, and explain them to your CA.

3. Give your patients financial options.

One of the biggest reasons that patients discontinue good care plans is money—not necessarily the lack of it, but the more complicated issues that arise when you don't straighten out all the financial details at the start when patients are giving you their best decisions and commitments.

Work out payment issues before beginning the report of findings. Explain to the patient all of their financial options.[1] I gener-

---

[1] I use and recommend Cash Practice (www.cashpractice.com) and like the three op-

ally suggest that practices finance or extend credit to patients so they can get the care they need and pay for it at their own pace.

4. Restate and recommit the patient to their care schedule and financial arrangements.

After the ROF, share your plan with your CA while the patient is still with you. This three-way agreement starts the administration of payment and appointment plans.

Let me explain why this is important: In the ROF, the patient hears about the care they need and how to pay for it. Then these concepts become concrete realities as the CA writes out all the details. If objections come up, the CA can handle them right there.

Exercise: This is easy—put together a hypothetical care and payment plan. In a training session with your staff, explain the appointment and payment plans of this hypothetical patient to your CA. The CA should then role-play their explanation of the appointment process, make the appointments, and go over the fine detail of the patient payment plan. At first, listen and comply, but as your CA gains expertise, increase the objections and work out rough spots.

5. Be genuinely glad to see your patients, and be interested in them.

There is nothing that can replace personal warmth and a sincere interest in your patients' well-being.

A doctor I know who specializes in difficult cases from all over the world mentioned that she goes through a lot of tissues at her office. I asked why. She told me she frequently cries with her patients when they become emotional about their problems. Her

tions that they give the patients. I love saying: "All options save you a good amount of money. I donâĂŻt care which one you choose. It all depends on what works best for you."

patients know she truly cares about them, and that's at least one reason why she virtually never loses a patient.

Exercise: Greet every patient with a "Good to see you, (name)." We all love to hear our own name, and everyone likes to be recognized, appreciated and approved of. Remember those classic scenes on *Cheers* when everyone would shout, "Norm!"

6. Help your patients focus on the importance of the next care goal.

Here you need to be a combination doctor, coach, and cheerleader. When the patient is in the relief phase, coach them on how to get to correction and how important that is. When they are in correction, coach on how to get the best correction, and move on to strengthening.

We are always focused on how to get to the next step and how important each step it. This is called leadership. It's essential for good compliance.

Exercise: Role-play conversations with a patient to explain the three phases of chiropractic care, tell them where they are, and talk about the importance of the next step.

7. Be quick to "come alongside" the patient to fix problems with appointments, care recommendations, or payment problems.

If a patient demonstrates a weak commitment to their care, express your concern. Don't bully people with a my-way-or-the-highway approach. Assume they want to do their best, but multiple factors may make it hard.

Here's something to say that can help you save a good patient from poor decisions and boost your patient compliance: "You're scaring me with how we're treating your appointments, Gina, and

I'm pretty brave. If I didn't mention it, I wouldn't be a good doctor, and neither of us wants that. Is there anything wrong?"

Exercise: Role-play with your CA "coming alongside" three patients you both know are having trouble keeping their appointments.

15

Building a Referral Practice

Would you like to know how to get an extra three to five new patient referrals every week? Of course you would! Everyone loves referrals. They come to the office already believing and ready to pay. They also make great patients.

So what do you need to do to double or triple your patient referrals this year? Follow these tips, and I promise you'll see more new patient referrals.

Envision your practice.

Referral Tip #1: Develop a strong vision for your practice, and then clarify, strengthen, and share it to increase referrals.

I've coached thousands of doctors over the last twenty-five-plus years. I've seen the successful become more so and the struggling grow by leaps and bounds. The doctors who've developed referral practices all have one thing in common—strong visions for their practices.

Exercise: Write your vision for your practice, preferably in under four hundred words, by answering the following questions:

- What is your chiropractic philosophy?
- What type of patients do you love to care for?
- Why do those types of patient respond so well to chiropractic?
- What do you want your office to look, sound, and feel like?
- What do you want a busy, productive hour in your practice to look like?
- What type of impact do you want to make on your community for health and chiropractic?

Share it with your staff and favorite patients. Insert portions into your report of findings, New Patient Orientation Class, and anywhere else it seems appropriate.

Say thank you.

Referral Tip #2: To encourage referrals, become an expert at the uncommon art of a sincere "thank you."

Good manners are in short supply here in the United States. There may be a worldwide shortage. What's been called common courtesy—a simple "thank you"—will stand out like a beacon and impress patients.

Exercise: Write sincere thank-you notes every week to:
1. Patients who referred a new patient to you (include a personal "P.S." for extra impact)
2. Business owners or managers for exceptional service
3. Patients who write chiropractic testimonies or give favorable online reviews
4. Businesses where you have done screenings

Prompt your patients to thank their referrer. When patients get excited about their chiropractic care, I ask them if they've thanked the friend who referred them: "Ann, have you told Paul how much better you're feeling? You might give him a call. I know he'd be pleased."

Create an upbeat, positive clinic.

Referral Tip #3: Make over your office decor and patient procedures to produce consistent quality in customer service and patient care.

I've seen thousands of chiropractic offices. What never fails to amaze me is how many of them need a makeover. Most aren't impressive—and I don't mean posh features like marble, leather, and original art on the walls. I mean spaces that are clean, bright, and attractive.

Makeovers don't stop with the interior design. Make sure your staff members are executing patient procedures with consistent quality.

Exercise: Make a template of a "perfect patient experience" in your clinic. It may include:

- Inspecting the outside for appearance (a freshly painted door and new brass hardware can make a world of difference)
- Cleaning, dusting, vacuuming, and throwing out the dead plant. Paint one wall an accent color, and hang every certificate you have
- Investing in uniforms for your CAs
- Training your staff to deliver an impressive greeting
- Running on time
- Practicing Day One, Day Two, the returning visit, reexam, and re-report, as well as New Patient Orientation classes with staff every month

Think of your practice as a great restaurant and you as the chef. Polish decor and performance to produce new patient referrals.

Collect patient testimonies.

Referral Tip #4: Collect patient testimonies.

I had just exited the exam room when my CA asked me if I could take another new patient. "Sure. Where did he come from?" I asked.

"Our reception room," she answered. "He's your current new patient's husband. He'd been reading the patient testimonies and found a story that was similar to his. He started asking some questions, and I told him you'd want to speak to him. I already have all his new patient paperwork."

Exercise: Collect patient testimonies, and structure them into three parts:

1. The problems the patient had before chiropractic
2. How the person came to be a chiropractic patient
3. How their life has changed for the better as a result of chiropractic

Keeping new patient testimonies in your reception or adjusting areas can be like having that patient sitting there all day telling their encouraging stories.

Just ask.

Referral Tip #5: Make a habit of artfully asking your patients to send you sick people to help.

A number of years ago, just after I'd bought a new luxury sedan, the salesman said, "I know you, Noel. You won't be able to keep your mouth shut about this car. Do me a favor. Tell 'em I've got more."

He was joking, but he also gave me three business cards with his mobile number underlined. I gave them to three friends, and I've given his name to at least a dozen others since. Why? When you're excited about something and like the people involved, it's a pleasure to refer them new business.

Exercise: Ask patients for referrals.

"Anita, Mandy tells me you're feeling better. How's your life improved since chiropractic?"

"That's fantastic. I never tire of hearing stories just like that. May I ask a favor?"

"I'm still accepting new patients, and I love referrals. Would you tell your story to someone who needs to know about chiropractic and give them this referral card? It's good for a free consultation."

My mindset is that I'm asking them to share some wonderful news, not telling them that I need the business.

Tell them why.

Referral Tip #6: Teach each new patient how chiropractic works in a New Patient Orientation class.

This may be a shock to you, but most patients can't explain what chiropractic is to their friends or family. Patients can't make an intelligent referral until they know how chiropractic works and what types of problems respond well to chiropractic care. You need to teach them.

Exercise: Construct, borrow, or buy a New Patient Orientation class program, and illustrate it with your own patient testimonies. Then put it into practice by:

- Requiring the class for all new patients, and scheduling them for it
- Starting your class at exactly the time you promised, and letting attendees go when promised
- Using your patients' true-life stories to illustrate each principle (patients love to hear about real successes)

Teach from the heart about the most wonderful healing art you know: chiropractic.

Put it all together.

Referral Tip #7: Assemble the first six tips on building a referral practice, and then practice, practice, practice. You will increase your new patient referrals.

A friend of mine took up golf last week, perfected his game over the last couple of days, and now shoots even par every round.

What? You don't believe me? Good for you—it isn't true. And here's just as big a fib: A friend of mine got six tips on how to build a referral practice and one week later sees five to eight referrals a week.

Every valuable skill takes time, practice, and determination to acquire.

Exercise: Track each of the six referral tips, practicing them daily until you master them, and produce a consistent stream of new patient referrals.

Here are a few more tips for pulling it all together:

- Teach each of the six referral tips to your CAs and colleagues.
- Place a list of the six referral tips in your office as a reminder that you'll see every morning.
- Each day, check off the referral tips that you worked on.
- Do not expect perfection—just work to make progress and be persistent.
- Do not give up or speak negatively to yourself if you lose focus or quit. Just get back at it.
- Do each of the referral tips until it becomes part of your daily practice habit. Good habits lead to a good life.

No one ever stimulated more patient referrals by just reading about them. In the same way, nobody ever got good at golf without practice and perseverance.

16

Getting Paid

I love to write advice on leadership, management, and what makes people tick, but this isn't about that.

This is a simple explanation of how to get more of your hard-earned money—real take-home cash—out of your accounts receivable (AR) and into your pocket, with the least amount of stress possible.

This is also not about insurance coding or packaging your services for maximum profitability. I'm not against a thoughtful approach to charging for what you do—we chiropractors typically give away more services than any health-care provider I know.

This chapter takes you step-by-step through a simple system that consistently rings 96 percent out of my AR year after year after year.

The back-story: I built ten clinics in a state with low insurance reimbursement and a practice scope that didn't allow most therapies. My charges per visit were a fraction of what chiropractors get in some states.

With more than one overhead to feed, I knew that if I billed it, I'd better collect it. So I developed a system for maximizing collections on services rendered.

If you don't think this subject applies to you, maybe you should take a closer look at your AR. If you extend credit to patients, I'll bet I can find $25,000 you should have collected last year.

I learned that the longer money was owed, the higher the chance that I wouldn't collect it. I also learned that uncollected money is not an orphan. Poor business practices and fear of confrontation are usually the not-so-proud parents.

And extra cash isn't the only by-product of taming your AR. You'll also have much lower stress. When you learn to face and handle any money problem, you cut your stress in half.

Before we begin, let me warn you the first couple of "sessions" can be a little harrowing. You may not be a "numbers person," or you may even resent that "a healer has to consider business." (Yes, that's an actual quote—guess what *that* DC's AR looked like).

I was forced to develop my collection system by need, but whatever your reasons are, you need to do it, and it will get easier.

This is how to do the Dirty Dozen—in other words, how to tackle the twelve worst accounts.

Step 1: Print a paper copy of an aged AR with patients in alphabetical order (not sorted by class or type such as personal injury). Include their current, 30-, 60-, 90-, 120-day, and total charges. Get the account start date, plus the date and amount of the last payment.

Why print it to paper? I know you bought that fancy computer that produces all those fancy reports on the promise that you could go paperless, right? But in this case, paper is your working copy that you will annotate. Do it on paper.

Step 2: Schedule your first 60-minute meeting with your CA. Eventually, these meetings will get shorter, and a lot more fun, than this first one.

Step 3: Explain to your CA that you're going to research each account in the entire aged AR, looking for the twelve worst accounts, based on three criteria: *size of balance*, *payment history*, and *security*.

> **Balance size:** It's obvious that if you're going to take action—such as billing, rebilling, phone calls, or collection proceedings—size matters. Look at the large dollar accounts first.
>
> **Payment history:** Any account that isn't being paid down according to your agreement should be investigated, put on watch, and maybe receive immediate attention.
>
> **Security:** If a personal injury case is being handled by a trusted attorney who's given a letter of protection, the $4,500 balance owed may be quite safe.

Step 4: You and the CA should go over the whole report—each account—looking at total amounts owed and deciding which are the twelve worst accounts. Look for big total balances, then the 90-day+ column for old money.

Don't stop to debate, argue, or work on one single account. Go through them all. Find the worst. You're only allowed to have twelve dirty accounts at the end. You'll get to the rest in time.

Why twelve? You can really only deal with one account at a time, and twelve seems to be the maximum you can handle in a week.

Step 5: Now pull all of the files on your four dirtiest accounts. Check the way the account was set up and open each of the computer ledgers. Were they billed correctly?

You're going to be amazed. Some accounts may have never been billed, some may be hung up in the electronic clearinghouse, some payments are "stuck" at the insurance company, and some may have been made but never posted to the account.

Step 6: Make assignments to bill, rebill, and call each dirty account. Get reports on your collection assignments **every day**—not yearly, monthly, or weekly, but **daily**. When the CA brings in the money, celebrate.

Step 7: This is where the Dirty Dozen becomes fun. After you've done the same thing, week after week, your CA can start leading you through a meeting that's now only thirty minutes long.

What do you have in the end? You and your CA know your AR like the back of your hands. You know where the money is, and you have all that lovely cash in your pocket.

A client started with $177,000 in AR when we began doing his Dirty Dozen meetings, and even with record production, they have only $55,000 today. That's an additional $127,000 profit for my client in just two years.

17

Problems in Your Practice

There's no shortage of problems in the day-to-day operation of a chiropractic practice—new or old, large or small. Everyone has problems. Chances are you're reading this to get some special insight on how to get rid of the problems in your own chiropractic practice.

But I think problems have gotten a bad rap. Every good thing I have came courtesy of a problem. I believe every problem has a solution, and it's discovering the solution—including the struggle—that excites me.

I can't think of one successful client who wasn't forced into positive change by a problem. And the single most important success strategy I know is how to reframe and deal with problems.

I want you to think differently about your chiropractic practice's problems. The following concepts will help.

1. **Realize that every doctor and every practice has problems—without exception.** You mustn't get discouraged by thinking that other DCs don't face the same challenges you do. It's also a mistake to believe you should have a breakthrough

where all of your problems disappear. You won't. Some DCs handle their difficulties better than others, and some have a better set of problems, but problems are universal. The happiest and most successful people I know frequently have the biggest problems. That's because they think about and approach problems differently.

2. **Be mindful that very few problems are accidents.** Rather, they're typically the collective result of decisions, actions, or lack of actions. Understanding this is key to taking responsibility for discovering a solution to your problems.

3. **They won't go away by focusing on them or ignoring them.** If you do either, the problems typically just get bigger.

A consulting client used to like to recite her problems to me. Unconsciously, she was trying to sell me on how reasonable her plight was in light of all her problems. The net effect was that she paralyzed herself with the gruesome picture she'd painted. When I told her we wouldn't talk about her problems ever again, she was horrified. However, that single step was the start of adding 125 patient visits a week to her practice.

4. **Reframing is an essential tool.** In order to handle your problems more effectively, you need think differently. When disaster strikes, you must know (at least intellectually) that the solution might be so spectacular that you will eventually be grateful for the setback. This will help you bypass your "Chicken Little" reflex as fast as possible and go as quickly as you can to a let-me-at-it mode to start solving the puzzle.

I was happily seeing more than four hundred patients a week, with associates seeing another 220 patients a week, when a career-ending ski accident turned my whole world upside down. At first I was devastated, but four years later, I was overseeing five clinics seeing two thousand visits a week. Out of that transformation, I developed Five Star Management. Thank you, Mr. Injury Problem.

Can you see how your current problem, even the biggest one, might be a future best friend?

5. **There are only a few real problems that practices face.** Actually, I've found there are only three. And if you aren't working on at least one of them, you're in trouble.

Right away many of you can think of at least a dozen problems affecting chiropractic practices, right? But I think that *real* problems are scarce. The way I do the math on what qualifies as a *real* problem is this: If I stumble in this area, my entire practice pays dearly. Conversely, if I solve one of these problems, then even though I may have other serious difficulties, my practice will improve dramatically.

So what's the biggest practice problem? Simple: *not enough new patients*, which should be no great surprise to you if you've read the previous chapters. If you get lots of new patients, you can be a mediocre chiropractor and have a wonderful practice. And if you're the best adjuster in the world, you won't succeed if your new patient "thing" is broken.

Numbers two and three are *poor retention* and *bad business systems*, respectively, but let's stick to new patients for now.

How does struggling terribly to bring in new patients ever get to be that "best friend" problem I mentioned earlier? In my case, I knew that new patients would always be a challenge, and so I opted for the best set of new patient problems I could find:

- *New patient problem #1:* In one month we produced 601 new patients for my five offices. I had seventeen full- and part-time staff, and that required scheduling, plus logistics challenges and costs.

- *New patient problem #2:* We opened a clinic that drew 161 new patients in one month. Believe me, it wasn't pretty, but it sure was exciting. There were days that the clinic looked like a bus rolling down a hill, with people flying everywhere.
- *New patient problem #3:* Last week, one of my clinics had twenty-eight new patient appointments scheduled, yielding twenty new patient show-ups. One day there were four new patients in reception at the same time, all filling out paperwork, and the regular patient schedule was full. Whew! We were packed and racked. Did it go smoothly? Not that day. Even though we're good and used to being busy, that day was a zoo.

Intensity and challenges aside, give me *this* set of new patient problems over the "who cut my phone lines and locked my door?" set of new patient problems any day!

18

Why Patients Stay for a Lifetime

"Jim, we've busted our tails going through relief, correction, and strengthening, and I'm proud of both of us."

"Me too."

"You know what most people do when they get to this point?"

"I know. They get a monthly checkup to stay healthy, right?"

"No, Jim. They fight like crazy to get right back down to where they started."

"You're kidding?"

"Wish I was. May I tell you what I'd like you to do instead?"

"I hope you will."

"Jim, welcome to the club."

Years ago, I was frustrated with the low number of maintenance and wellness patients my practice had. There were a few but not enough by my liking. Plus, smart people who owed everything to chiropractic were frequently nowhere to be found.

For a fresh perspective on my missing maintenance patients, I hired a public opinion research company to study the problem. And after spending lots of time and money, what I discovered was disturbing.

"First, Dr. Lloyd, you have the highest-rated business we've ever measured. Your patients are very satisfied. Second, they don't think they need any more care."

I was livid. "That's impossible! I tell them, then I tell what I told them again."

"Dr. Lloyd, the research is clear, and I'm just telling you what they told us."

I didn't like that answer, but I had to believe it. However, I was going to get to the bottom of this. Since I'd already asked the "lost" why they strayed, now I'd ask the committed why they stayed.

We asked some of our best patients, "Are you a lifetime chiropractic patient?" A good number said they were, and I set up interviews with eight of them. What I learned was priceless, and it literally doubled my retention.

The entire group had received monthly checkups for at least three years and had been under care for at least ten years. Half were insurance, and half paid cash. No one was wealthy. Six of the eight had tried to live without chiropractic and couldn't.

Like so many chiropractic offices, we had dozens of patients who used chiropractic for crisis care, sometimes over decades, but as wonderful as these folks were, I was looking to learn from those who didn't need pain as a motivator.

The following is my report on what my real-life lifetime patients taught me and how you can help others use chiropractic like we do—for maintenance and wellness. Here we go:

All of the patients were educated in chiropractic. Each one could explain how chiropractic worked and understood subluxation or "nerve pressure." They knew they could skip a correction and not feel it initially, but it was "bad juju," as one man put it, and *that* was why he got checked before any symptoms showed up.

They agreed that everyone should be at least checked for subluxation and that subluxation caused nerve energy to be strangled and caused "almost anything."

They were believers. Each had their own story, but the result was the same—they believed.

With the war raging for the hearts and minds of people everywhere to put their faith in medicine, drugs, and surgery, we need true believers in chiropractic.

One man parroted a phrase I taught him: "I believe in chiropractic first, drugs second, surgery last." Amen, brother!

They all had a good relationship with great DCs and CAs. We've all heard that people buy the messenger before they buy the message, right? I'm feeling a bit immodest here, but remember, these people rated our clinic sky high for customer service. Translation? They knew we loved them and put their interests first.

They had good results. Each one found that chiropractic was the best and only way to live healthily. Everyone loved their adjustments and, as one woman put it, "I CAN'T miss my monthly adjustment."

They had enough money. Remember, none of these folks were very well off, but all made sure they had enough for their chiropractic care. Not one person got any discounts on our reasonable adjustment prices.

Okay, now how do we activate these five common elements in patients today to produce real, lifetime chiropractic patients? Here's what I did:

1. In the report of findings, speak about relief, correction, strengthening, and maintenance of health as the goal from the start—and always point the way to the next level.

2. Make your New Patient Orientation class a conversion experience, where people are preached to and hear great testimonies of miraculous recoveries.

3. Train DCs and CAs on great customer service in everything you do. A full 67 percent of customers leave a company because of poor customer service.

4. Work on your technique. Never forget that great chiropractic technique gets the best results. My friend Jeff Ricks is going for his Part Three NUCCA certification at age sixty-four. Keep pushing.

5. Don't price yourself out of the market, but don't cheapen what we have to offer with discounts.

19

The Secrets of the Survivors

There were two signs in the window. The first read "Family Chiropractic Center," and the second, "Now for Lease: Call Ace Commercial Real Estate Brokerage."

Just a quick peek inside told the story: great colors, nice new carpet, fresh paint, interesting design detail in the front desk CA station, efficient central hall design…and a stack of letters on the floor under the mail slot—many with "FINAL NOTICE" stamped on the front.

A failed chiropractic business. Notice I didn't say a failed chiropractic *practice*. I would guess that the few patients the doctor saw were thrilled with the care. That's the way it is with chiropractic practices. Chiropractic works miracles, even for ordinary chiropractors. But it's the business of chiropractic that needs to prosper in order for the practice to survive.

If you're a chiropractic student, go back and read the previous sentence two more times, and remember it. If you've been in practice for a year or more, you can't forget it.

This doctor's misfortune illustrates that the science, art, and philosophy of chiropractic fails if the business of chiropractic fails. These three cherished components vanish from that office, that part of the community, that practice (the patients in care), and, in some cases, that doctor.

Try spending $150,000 on your chiropractic education and practice setup, and then tell your spouse and family that the money is gone, you can't pay your bills, and you're looking for work in construction. Would that test *your* faith?

"Yeah, chiropractic's great. It's just me that sucks." Ouch.

I'm so compelled by sympathy for chiropractors who are too close to that same fate that I have to say, and say emphatically, that it doesn't have to be that way. I've coached many chiropractors who turned to me for help in the eleventh hour who have been able to pull the nose up just before a disastrous crash and then have gone on to make a soaring success of their chiropractic business and practice. They found out that the difference between "died and gone to heaven" and "just plain dead" is knowing how to run a chiropractic business and running it well.

In the capitalist economy we have in the United States, the vast majority of health care is provided by private businesses. These private businesses, or practices, have to make a profit in order to survive. In chiropractic, that is even more so.

Like every other business, in chiropractic, there is the initial struggle to get, and then keep, a safe distance between total receipts and expenses—the difference being your net profit. If there's enough profit in your chiropractic practice, you can afford to provide services again next month, next year, and the year after that. In fact, if there's enough profit in your practice, your business model may be worthy of reproduction, but that's another discussion.

Since we are talking about profit, let's remind ourselves of the dreams that profits fund—you know, the wonderful house, nice cars, vacations, college for the kids, and a comfortable transition from full-time practice to part-time. (This is an end-game point here, but the happiest senior chiropractors I know still have their hands in practice one or two days a week. After all, they've spent decades building these skills and patient relationships; they're not just going to sit around and watch the dog.)

Here's an interesting fact about the purity of business evolution: the principle of "only the strong survive" is true in spades in the United States, where four out of five nonformatted businesses (we'll discuss formatted vs. nonformatted) die within five years. Lack of profit is always on the death certificate, and that's right, 80 percent die.

What did the other 20 percent do to succeed, you ask? Some don't know. That group can't take the credit; it was either dumb luck or natural talent. I've seen a lot of both, and neither can be replicated. They aren't the teachers. Teachers didn't know at first but learned—and now are kicking ass. Here's what they teach:

1. **Before you even start, vow to do whatever is necessary to succeed.** The only constraints on what you do should come from good ethics, and those guidelines are in the Golden Rule: do to others what you would have them do to you. A great ethics assessment for selecting your action steps is this: Would you want a chiropractor to use those action steps to acquire and treat your parents as patients?
2. **Never give up.** After honesty, determination is worth ten times any other attribute you can name.
3. **Embrace the fact that your practice is a start-up business.** Do whatever you need to do to learn and excel at the fundamentals of the business of chiropractic, which include the following:

Marketing: Everything else can be wrong, but if you're producing lots of new patients, you will make it. Everything else can be right, but if you're producing too few new patients, you will fail. This is a hard truth for some, but chiropractic requires sales, and chiropractors are salespeople.

Every business is sales, and everyone on the planet is a salesperson. Anyone who has an opinion is a salesperson. Decide to like it and to be very good at it. And remember that the sale doesn't end when someone becomes a patient, or when they choose lifetime care. It never ends.

If now you're saying to yourself, "I didn't get into chiropractic to be a salesperson. I'm a doctor, not a salesperson," let me set you straight. You have a self-image problem, or a fear of rejection, and you're trying to hide behind a title or degree. If you can get over that, you'll succeed. If you can't, that may be your office in the first paragraph.

Management: You have three management challenges. Let's discuss the toughest first, because it's you. Your biggest management challenge is getting yourself to do whatever's needed to make your practice flourish. I'm not talking about slave-driving yourself through distasteful drudgery but artfully helping yourself build a love for doing what you need to do in order to build the practice of your dreams. It is the most challenging, rewarding, and worthy of all endeavors.

Your second management challenge is your staff. You may not have any staff at first, but you will. This will be the easiest of the three groups and therefore is often neglected. Few DCs invest the proper time, effort, and money in developing their staff. However, CAs, when properly trained and cared for, are the most consistent good in any chiropractic practice (and that includes the chiropractor).

The third management challenge is your chiropractic patients. Your objective here must be to be of value to and stay in a relationship with your patients for the rest of their lives. There isn't one person on the planet who doesn't need to have access to (and know and understand why they should see) their personal chiropractor.

For me, it boils down to this: if some other chiropractor were responsible for my family, I would want them to bring my wife and two boys through any relief, correction, and strengthening care possible and then into a lifetime chiropractic care program that included at least monthly checkups. Now, how to do this professionally for as many people as you care to and can serve is another lifetime challenge. But the good news is that just a few hours a week can make this a living reality.

Operations: This includes all of the mechanics of your business/practice, including the office and how it operates. Operations gets little attention, and that neglect produces so much stress.

An interesting case study in operations is the University of Washington Husky Marching Band. They do a great halftime show. Ever wonder how that show got so great? Practice, practice, practice. That's the essence of operations. However, less than one percent of all chiropractors actually practice their procedures "off the playing field." Ask Tiger Woods and Mark McGwire about practice.

Finance: In short, don't spend it until you have it. I know that's a little like locking the door after the horse has been stolen if you're $100,000 in debt to school loans, but if that's the case, it's even more important to be frugal. Start your practice with used furniture, used equipment, and a small office. Maybe rent space with an established DC who has all that already. After you start making money, get out of debt as fast as you can and especially before you buy that boat.

All right, that's the wake-up call. What do you do now, you ask? Three things:

First, believe. Believe that you can not only survive and succeed but you can have a blast doing it. It's like golf—the better your game gets, the more fun it becomes.

Second, get some help. Where did this Marlboro Man, Frank Sinatra-style "I Did It My Way" thing come from? Pros get help, but rookies are sometimes too proud/scared/dumb (take your pick). There are more out-of-business chiropractors because of this than anything else. Stop and ask for directions.

Third, hang in there. It's a journey. Some are further away from the goal than others, but "died and gone to heaven" often starts just a few steps past the point when you think you're "just plain dead."

20

No "Tu Fu Nu" for You

The story line is as old as time. A starry-eyed kid gets the crazy idea to really make a difference for good and, while battling the odds and pursuing the dream, finally has to face the bully in a fight where *everything's* at stake.

The struggle causes the kid to wonder whether they have what it takes for success. Riddled with self-doubt, they worry they'll let everyone down and fold up like a wet paper bag, spilling everything they have worked for onto the street in one big mess.

Then, at just the right moment, the kid hears somebody say, "Hey, it's just your entire life and everything you've ever dreamed of and worked for. No pressure."

Pretty dramatic, right? This might surprise you, but as a chiropractic practice coach, I run into this on a regular basis. It's all there: dreams, desires, struggles, fears, real danger, courage, and triumph. Sometimes the stories include the tragedy of broken dreams and loss.

Quite honestly, it's pretty exciting stuff. In my job, I root for the heroes and heroines every day. I get mentally and emotionally involved in what and who they care about. I tense up when things get scary—and they *do* get scary.

Insert your favorite movie title here, but since this is real life, chiropractic coaching is *better* than a movie. Still, let me make my point as if I'm pitching a movie to a film producer in some overpriced, snooty restaurant in West Hollywood. Ready? Follow closely now.

Here's the pitch:

> "Okay, we've got a young kid, somewhere between thirteen and sixteen years old (a young Brad or Angie, Toby or Kristen—doesn't matter) who has a life-changing experience with chiropractic, courtesy of the old neighborhood DC (think Christopher Lloyd in *Back to the Future*).
>
> "The DC spouts all that philosophy stuff and practices because he loves it and people need him. He's driven by what he knows about chiropractic. We'll call him 'Doc.'
>
> "Doc tells the kid he or she could be a chiropractor, too, and really help people. The kid's stunned 'Me? Really?' They lie awake nights, fantasizing about it.
>
> "The kid goes off to chiro school and into a zillion dollars of debt. Hey, let's throw the grandparents in here. They mortgage their house to help the kid. The kid's smart, studies hard, and gets out of school with the national and state board exams successfully passed.
>
> "The kid gets a break on a small, modest office that doesn't need much remodeling. In the script, the kid's dad helps with the build out. You see it? The whole

family is in on this—everyone's pulling for the kid. The audience will love it.

"Now comes the romance and the tension. If our kid's a guy, his girlfriend is being pestered by a third-year med student who keeps asking her when she's going to give up on the 'loser quack chiropractor' boyfriend. (You really hate this guy.)

If our young DC's a girl, we'll give her the same jerk med student guy! It's perfect! Everyone hates him right away. He wants to know when she'll give up on that loser quack garbage chiropractic. The audience will be yelling at the screen, 'Dump that creep!'

"Okay, the small open house that Mom catered before the practice's grand opening is just clearing out as Dad walks by the appointment book. He looks but sees no patients except the family. Dad asks the kid where the new patients come from, and the kid looks scared. 'They never taught that in school.'

"Then this evil-looking guy walks in to the kid's new office and says, 'You don't know how to get any new patients, do you? I'm going to close you down, kid. You'll go broke, lose all your family's money, and end up cleaning carpets at night for your brother-in-law!' Then he says, 'Allow me to introduce myself.' And just like a supervillain straight out of a Bruce Lee movie, he offers his name as Tu Fu Nu—that is, too few new patients (evil laugh here)."

Too melodramatic for you? Sorry, but it's my movie, and this is the concept I've been playing with for years. More great chiropractors get beaten up by not having enough new patients than anything else I know. That's why I've given this problem a name: "too few new" (Tu Fu Nu).

So how does the movie end? The kid goes to Doc, who got him or her interested in chiropractic in the first place. Doc's advice is good: "Honestly, kid, it's different today than when I started. You need to do everything from Internet to screenings to talks—everything. But you need to *learn* this stuff, not just wing it."

The kid decides, then and there, to learn to get the chiropractic message out of heart, head, and office and into the community. No matter what it takes! And THAT's when the excitement starts.

By the way, did I tell you there's a sequel?

Star in your own movie. Learn to kick Tu Fu Nu's butt, and your reality will be more fun than any fantasy.

Part Two

Have More Fun

Taking Care of Yourself

21

Choosing Chiropractic for Life

It took me sixteen years to make this decision, but believe me, it's a great one. I met my first chiropractor as a sick and scared four-year-old. I didn't like him or any of my first appointment much, but on the ride home after my first adjustment, my dad knew I was going to get well.

"I think we've got our son back," he told my mom.

A year prior, I had taken a serious fall, injuring my neck. My health took a bad turn, and I stayed sick, off and on, for an entire year. Eventually a friend of the family cornered my mother in a grocery store and begged her to take me to a chiropractor. My parents were desperate, so they did. Thank you, God.

My recovery was miraculous, and because of that, my parents were ready to learn all about chiropractic and accept what they were taught. My entire extended family started chiropractic care, and migraines, stomach problems, and poor health in general went away. What we learned about chiropractic, we believed and knew was true. Chiropractic was good for life.

I decided at age eleven to become a chiropractor. By the time I showed up at Palmer College, I had already spent hundreds of hours in chiropractic reception rooms, waiting for dozens of chiropractic adjustments. The results of those adjustments proved again that chiropractic was good for life.

Halfway through my training at Palmer College, sixteen years after my first trip to a chiropractor, I put the pieces together and made one of the most important decisions of my life. Here it is:

To be healthy I need a 100 percent connection with the life-giving, healing power of my Innate Intelligence (resident in my brain) flowing through my body.

My fall at age four hurt that connection by causing a subluxation (vertebra putting pressure on nerves) in my neck. I regained my health when the subluxation was corrected.

Over time, I was subluxated again, got sick again, went to the chiropractor again, and got healthy again. Because of what I know and because I want to live up to my best potential, I decided that I need to live subluxation free and that I would never again go any longer than a month without a chiropractic checkup and adjustment.

It's been more than forty years since I made that decision, and without a doubt, I can say that my commitment to regular chiropractic care is why I stand before you, healthy and enjoying my life. I invite you to join me in choosing chiropractic for life.

22

Thirteen Steps to a More Powerful You

The most powerful people in the world are those who can produce and control strong positive emotions, and you can learn their secrets.

Think about it. The power to produce excitement, optimism, belief, power, and enthusiasm can be right at your fingertips, or even closer—right between your ears! Gives you goose bumps, doesn't it?

What follows is my personal recipe for developing that type of power, control, and enthusiasm.

Use this thirteen-step action plan to take your life from drudgery to dynamic and from blah to BOOM in as few as ten days!

I promise that if you pick just three to five of the following proven tips, you'll be on your way to reprogramming yourself to show up strong and excited where and when you need it the most.

1. **Get up early, even if you don't feel like it.** A new day is a metaphor, and excited people want to grab the new day when

it's young, not hide from it under the covers. Learn to love the early morning. I get two or three hours of solitude and time to tinker with my head before my busy life and commitments rush in to meet me. *Early riser trick: Turn off the TV long before the evening news, and read something inspirational before you go to bed.*

2. **Eat protein in the morning.** Diet plays a huge part in your mood, and you know your own blood sugar, so balance it. Think this way: "I'll eat for how I want to feel, not just for taste." I put down two eggs by 4:30 a.m. every morning before I go to work out.

3. **When you get up, go exercise.** At least take a brisk walk. The increased endorphins, muscle tone, and positive body image will push you physically and emotionally in the right direction. Plus, your exercise time is a great time to listen to and speak your positive affirmations.

   FYI #1: Successful and enthusiastic people get their lives in control. It's been decades since I first heard the phrase "good habits, good life," but I've never found an exception to that rule. Get your morning mastered, and you're on your way to true power and excitement.

   FYI #2: Successful and enthusiastic people also know that they frequently have to take the right action before the feelings of excitement or power show up. Think this way: "Fake it until you make it!"

4. **On your way to work, listen to positive, affirming music.** If you're alone, sing your brains out. Anything from Journey's "Don't Stop Believin'" to the hymn "How Great Thou Art" will raise your spirits. *Another good commute tip: Reflect on and relive the best contributions individual staff members have made to your practice. It will make seeing them a real pleasure, and pleasure = excitement.*

5. **Get to the office early and lead your team in a "mini-pump" session around the appointment book.** Take turns reading at least part of your chiropractic statement of purpose, then give sincere compliments to staff. Continue to recognize their contributions throughout the day.

6. **Greet each patient enthusiastically.** Talk louder but use fewer words, and focus on chiropractic—not symptoms, politics, gossip, or anything negative.

7. **Write or rewrite your affirmations, and read them again late in the day.**

8. **Share patient progress with staff and other patients through oral, written, and online testimonies.** Put several patient testimony books in your reception area, always open to an exciting chiropractic recovery. I have also collected twelve patient testimonies in a private binder that I keep at my desk to review when I need it.

9. **Keep your practice clear of negative materials.** See how many drug ads there are in the weekly trash rags? Don't let them into your space. Stay off the Internet (including Twitter and Facebook) and avoid texting your friends about non-chiropractic garbage. Present-time consciousness produces more new patients than social media.

10. **Attend technique seminars.** Better technique means better chiropractors doing better chiropractic *and* getting better chiropractic results. If that's not exciting, what is?

11. **Attend philosophy meetings and seminars.** Challenge your mind with new ideas and inspirational speakers. And offer your own philosophy seminars in your New Patient Orientation classes, sharing positive testimonies and the broader story of chiropractic.

12. **Associate only with positive DCs and CAs.** Dump your negative chiropractor buddies. "Wow, Noel. That's cold.

These guys are my friends." Really? People who try to recruit you to their fears by sharing their doom and gloom are just trying to drag you down. Don't let them!

13. **Attend seminars where you get motivated, encouraged, and built up.** That's where you'll find your new DC and CA friends.

Everyone wants to be excited and carried to new heights on the wings of enthusiasm. Yet strong, positive emotions start with our determination and commitment.

A friend said, "You're lucky, Noel. You're passionate about what you do." I'm blessed, but every day I also make at least a hundred decisions to live—not perfectly, but consistently inside these disciplines.

Now, pick three or five or seven of these actions, and hold yourself joyfully accountable to establish the habits. They'll produce all the power you'll ever need. Here's to your success!

23

Focus

I love being focused, and it's my guess that you do too. That alert, clear-headed feeling, where you're catching things on the fly and making good decisions quickly, is exciting. Even now, in my sixties, being focused makes me feel like a kid. Present-time consciousness, passion, and confidence are all first cousins of focus, which turns work into a game. Focus is the optimal way to work and live.

When you're out of focus, you're bored, confused, and distracted. We can blame a ton of chiropractic practice woes on a lack of focus. In fact, most of the stress that's created by allowing important issues to slip through the cracks comes from a problem with focus.

Does sharp focus come to only a select few, like a random gift, leaving others wanting? Is the intense attention to important issues that is the hallmark of focus the accident of genetics, dumb luck, or the result of a series of conscious decisions and actions? No. We can all learn how to keep our focus through trials and avoid boredom or distraction.

Twenty-five-plus years of coaching experience tells me that when we are in control of our thoughts, we can all learn how to enjoy more and be more successful.

Most doctors who have learned to focus their attention and energies have a couple tricks up their sleeves that keep them focused. Here are a few of mine:

1. Have vision, goals, and action.

Focus springs naturally and effortlessly from a clear vision, specific goals, and effective action. I ask my consulting clients to visualize what they want and tell me what it looks like. Then we break that down into specific daily, weekly, and monthly goals. That will take them from wishing to reality. And effective action moves me from where I am to my vision and goal.

Exercise: Write out your vision for your practice, preferably in fewer than four hundred words. Then write out your specific goals for new patients, established patients, production, collections, and patient visit average. Now check your vision and goals against reality and find out where to apply your focus.

Example: One of my clinics had a so-so kept appointment average (KAP) of 84 percent—not my vision or my goal of at least 92 percent. We focused on specific actions to fix our KAP and saw it increase to 93 percent. We saw what we wanted, set a goal, and took the action.

2. Use checklists.

Everyone who knows me knows I love checklists. A checklist is written focus.

I learned about the value of checklists while learning to fly airplanes more than forty years ago. Each item on an aviation checklist represents a mistake someone previously made in an environment that requires no mistakes just to stay alive.

You can map out the best procedures for the practice you envision and put them in a checklist so you hit your goals.

Example: It's been brought to your attention that patients aren't being greeted the way you want at the front desk. Create a checklist that outlines each step of the greeting: standing, smiling, the welcome script, etc. Then practice the checklist with your staff until it's done perfectly. This is the very process of being focused.

3. Surround yourself with focused people.

Spend your time with people who share your vision and your goals. One of the things I love about my consulting clients is that they've each agreed to push themselves and each other on their practice visions and goals and to take specific action to produce a best-ever year in their practices.

Do whatever is necessary to be in that type of company.

4. Practice, practice, practice.

Focus is a skill and takes practice. For years, I would start my practice day reviewing the Daily Dozen, a set of twelve attitudes and actions that I wanted to incorporate in my behavior—some as simple as deciding to be positive every time I entered a room. There were days that I would hit everything on my list for a couple hours straight. Other days, I'd stumble in the first twenty minutes. However—and here's the key—instead of giving up when I slipped, I'd go back to my checklist and see if I could stay focused longer next time. The more I practiced focus, the more focused I became. It's that simple.

Another discipline that's been worth its weight in gold is the conscious decision to leave my problems outside, on the azalea by the back door, when I enter the clinic. It is my focused desire and disciplined choice to make my practice a refuge, not only for the patients and the staff but also for me. It is so much easier to focus on the tasks at hand when my personal problems are left to wait outside on the shrub.

5. Apply the Swiss watch perspective.

There are few things as beautiful as the workings of a Swiss watch. The precision, craftsmanship, and product (keeping accurate time) is a work of art. That same beauty can be seen in your practice if you craft your vision, set your goals, and take action to make your practice a work of art. I have coached hundreds to the Swiss watch standard, and they tell me this concept has helped their focus.

6. Focus on the big picture.

Why bother with any of this? We have one life, and each of us has the rest of that life to live by choice. We are not victims. We have an obligation to focus our dreams, ideas, and energies on our practices and build them the way we want them to be.

If you don't teach patients how to be good, happy citizens of your practice, who will? And if you do, what a great practice you will have.

24

Creating Power Hours

I like asking chiropractors what they enjoy most about their practice. It offers me an insight into the person, and it typically starts an enjoyable conversation.

The most common answer I hear is a description of the time when the house is packed, the energy is upbeat, and the doctor's "in the zone," going from one table or room to the next. They're confident, having fun, taking great care of patients, and hearing about their progress. I call these times power hours.

During a conversation with a seminar guest, he told me that "those [power hour] times are all too rare. I wish it could be like that all the time."

"I think I can help with that," I said, as I called a client over to join the conversation. After introductions, I said, "Tell our guest about your power hours." My client's eyes lit up as he described his busiest, highest energy, and most enjoyable hours in the clinic.

"Power hours used to happen by accident, but then Noel showed me how to plan for and create them. Now there are four times as many power hours in the practice as when we started," he said.

"That makes practice a lot more fun, doesn't it?" said our seminar guest.

"It's better than that. We added 120 visits a week and cut our stress in half, all due to power hours."

I was quick to add that it also took thought, planning, and discipline to make the change, but my client was just as quick to say that it was well worth the effort—times ten!

My guest looked straight at me and said, "If I get this one thing and nothing else out of the weekend, it'll be worth the trip. Will you teach me what you taught your client?"

"I'd be happy to," I said.

The following is what I told him, and if you want to help more people, have more fun, and make better money using power hours, read on.

First, let's get our thinking straight. The best thing that chiropractors can do for their patients is find and remove subluxations, and that doesn't take very long.

How long does it take to adjust your spouse, kids, or best friend? Probably not very long, and that tells you something about your real adjustment time. Much of the time a patient spends in your office is lost to lack of training for staff, doctor, and patient, as well as off-purpose socializing—chatting about the weather, sports, your upcoming vacation, or the patient's new car. When the exchange degenerates into chitchat, you're not only wasting time, but you're ruining the doctor-patient relationship.

Patients want you focused on chiropractic and them.

Find out how many patients you can see in an hour by asking your CA to time your next office call. I'm not advocating that you rush people through—never rush your technique—but don't lollygag either. Find the time that reflects your style.

There is no judgment here about the outcome, just feedback. You don't want to over- or under-book your power hours. The goal is to replicate the pace you get when you are "in the zone." We'll call this your *power hour rate*.

Reality check: Before you ask your CA to time you, ask them how many patients they feel comfortable booking for you in an hour. If you know you can do great work on ten to twelve (or more) patients an hour and the CA says five or six, they may be telling you that you waste time.

Now select the three busiest hours you currently have, pack them at capacity based on your power hour rate, and create your first three power hours.

The key to effective power hours is to stay disciplined by following the rules.

First, stay on purpose, on task, and on time. And second, only do adjustments. Book all of your other procedures at other times.

One of the big enemies of staying on time is the temptation to overadjust too many segments, too many times. When a patient says, "I don't think you got it, Doc," assure them you did, smile, and confirm their next appointment.

When you learn to create and perfect a power hour, you're primarily training yourself, but you're also training your patients and your staff. When you get really good at doing a power hour, your CA and your patients will enjoy the time, too One of my clients, who practices in a large, fast-paced city, tells me that his patients request power hour appointments by name because they know they can get in and out on time.

Reality check: You may be thinking, "I have patients who came from a big practice up the road, and they tell me they left that practice because the doctor didn't spend enough time with them." I've heard that, too, typically from a patient who wants to train me to spend a lot of unnecessary time rubbing this, checking that, or trying to get me to adjust something again. Frankly, I'd rather have the big practice up the road and have those people see someone else.

Now the game starts: Work with your CA to see how many power hours you can schedule in a week. Regularly ask your staff questions like: *How are my times? How would you grade our power hours? How's the energy in the office during power hours?*

When the new power hours fill up, add more. Set a goal to add one to two new power hours a week.

And remember that creating power hours allows you to give better care, help more people, have more fun, make more money, feel a higher sense of purpose, and demonstrate better leadership and organization. Plus, by guiding patients toward power hours, it leaves other time slots open for more new patients!

25

Getting the Mechanics Right

Headspace is the key, right? It's mind over matter, isn't it?

Not this time.

Hank Haney, golf coach to top pros and celebrities, has a reality program on TV called *The Haney Project*. Hank has coached the best in the game, including Tiger Woods. But in his TV show, he takes a celebrity with a terrible game and tries to fix it. He looks for interesting personalities, like Charles Barkley and Rush Limbaugh, as his "projects." It's a smart formula that produces entertaining TV, even if you don't like golf.

I like this show because of the similarities to my own work. I'm a DC who built a clinic system with eight associates and two thousand patient visits per week. I'm also a coach who's mentored some of the top chiropractors around the world. Like Haney, I've had some very challenging "project" clients who took every ounce of skill I possessed. But when a project goes well, it's beautiful.

A growing list of these clients who started out as projects have transformed before my eyes, increasing their practices by one hundred to three hundred patient visits a week. Many go on to sustain that growth, and an increasing number become my dream clients, staying for many years and focusing on new challenges and exciting solutions.

When I speak of my project clients' breakthroughs, the smart people in the room ask me to name the single most important change that allowed their extraordinary growth. That's a great question.

In one of The Haney Project episodes, Rush Limbaugh asks Hank about the mental part of the game of golf. Haney responds, "Get the mechanics right, and the mental takes care of itself."

In other words, if you pound the ball 280 yards off the tee and drop it in the middle of the fairway then hit it tight to the pin from 174 yards out, your mental game will follow. I love that clarity.

Here's why this is so important to you and me and is also the key to how I've helped my project clients: get the mechanics of a great practice right, and you'll be successful.

Guess what follows? That's right, the mental part of the game— what many call head space.

A pet peeve of mine is that so many practice coaches frustrate their clients by blaming their headspace for their lack of success.

For example, the client says, "My number of new patients is down, and my practice is crashing." The weak coach replies, "It's your headspace." What does that even mean? If you think a certain way, do new patients float into your office on the vapors created by your headspace?

The headspace answer is a catch-all, a BS dodge for a weak coach who doesn't know how to help their client.

I understand why a weak coach blames headspace—it puts the ball in the client's court—but the answer is perfectly useless. It can also make the client feel like they have an inferior chiropractic philosophy. Surely, the doctor in the busy, successful practice has a good headspace.

That's usually true, but it doesn't explain where that healthy stream of new and returning patients came from. In the thousands of practices I've coached, this is the key: **successful doctors have good mechanics**.

I think Haney's answer is the real truth. Get the mechanics right, and the mental (confidence) will follow.

As I've shared before, I once produced 601 new patients in a one-month period for my own clinics. Additionally, I opened a new clinic that attracted 161 new patients in the first month. My headspace was great, but it was my mechanics that created the appeal to new patients.

I learned several external marketing systems, and I worked them into templates with a series of steps that I could teach others. I hired assistants and trained them to replicate my marketing templates. I quickly found out who was productive and reliable. The super-reliable staff became my managers, with training and responsibility to hire their own assistants. We trained on my templates relentlessly, usually on the job. We kept the good ones and quickly said goodbye to the bad.

To stay in control of the mechanics, I developed a system where all my marketing managers and assistants reported to me every day on good *and* bad news. I was never out of touch. My biggest clinic launch was handled by a twenty-four-year-old woman named Jodi, who I had trained. She hired and trained the team that produced 161 new patients the first month the practice was open. Another manager oversaw the group of marketing assistants, including my associates, who produced 601 new patients in one month. I did so little of the front-line work it's laughable.

The mechanics of a great golf swing haven't changed since Bobby Jones almost one hundred years ago. A grandmother with reasonable athletic ability who masters the mechanics of that swing will beat 95 percent of today's golfers.

When you know that you know what you're supposed to know, you feel good about walking up to the tee and can hardly wait to get into the office on Monday.

26

Get Kicked Out

I'll never forget the day I got kicked out of Trafalgar Square in London.

My colleague George Birnbach and I were taping a short video promo for our company, Five Star Management, when a warden—that's what it said on her badge—told us we had to have a permit to do a video.

"What about that man taping his kids?" I said.

She said, "That's different."

Still not sure what we were doing wrong, we moved across the street and completed the shot.

Looking back, I consider it a badge of honor that we were told to leave a public landmark like Trafalgar. (Besides, we already had shot we wanted.)

The whole encounter reminds me of one of my favorite sayings, "It's better to ask for forgiveness than permission." In other words, don't worry about what might happen; just go for it. You'll get a lot more done.

It also reminds me of some rogue spinal screenings we've done—like the time we set up a SAM at an event where there were people who needed to know about chiropractic, without getting any special permit or permission.

We screened on a busy public street another time. Hey, we're the public, right? We thought that we might run into a little trouble, but we just went for it. We met a few great new patients and packed up an hour later with no incident.

It felt a little like when we were kids, ringing the neighbors' doorbell and running, or throwing snowballs at cars—exciting and a bit risky, but not hurtful.

The person who gives others the power to rule over their actions, or is worried about what people think, or is always looking for permission from some outside authority figure is generally too scared to have any fun or break free.

That reminds me of another favorite saying, "No risk, no reward, no exception." Break free. Go for it.

27

Get Excited!

It's easy to find yourself feeling demotivated, especially if you've been at this for a while, doing the same things over and over. You feel stuck, and it's almost like you have a writer's block feeling about how to move your practice forward.

If that sounds familiar, here are some tips that always get me reinspired.

Relearning What I Already Knew

I like the morning. I'm generally up early to eat a small breakfast, drink my coffee, check the morning news, and then I'm off to the health club. I sit outside at 5:10 a.m., checking my email and waiting for the club to open.

Once I'm inside, I fire up a podcast or start listening to an audiobook, and suddenly my mind is racing around dozens of ideas and concepts—some new, but many familiar. It's like reconnecting with a good friend you've almost forgotten but are happy to see again.

Before I know it, the thirty-six minutes on the StairMaster are over. Where did the time go? Once again, I've tricked my body during what might be a boring-beyond-endurance activity by sending my brain on a wonderful excursion through a great author's thoughts.

Great thought and exercise are old friends. My late father-in-law, John McDiarmid, spent time at the Institute for Advanced Study in New Jersey. My wife, just a little girl at the time, remembers the professors walking all over the town. Her mother explained that the exercise helped them think. Today iPods, iPhones, and every other MP3 player on the market allows us to listen to the great and inspiring thoughts of others while we burn off calories and pump up our pecs. What a deal!

Eighty minutes into my workout, I feel great, both physically and mentally. I've stopped several times between sets and reps to email myself an idea that bubbled to the surface while listening to wonderful, smart people read their inspiring words to me.

So load up your MP3 player with a couple of great books. I recommend *The E-Myth Revisited* by Michael Gerber, *Personal Accountability* by John G. Miller, or the biblical book of Second Corinthians by Paul, and stomp your local StairMaster into submission. Everybody wins.

The Right Answer

Ever been stumped by a patient question or objection and later wished you had done a better job with the answer? I meet doctors all the time who repeatedly struggle with that issue every day—how will they know the best answer? Many are stressed and live in a low-grade fear of those difficult questions coming up, and that can take a lot of the fun out of practice. If you collect enough of those issues, the practice is no fun at all.

If this ever happens to you, I have a solution for you.

Write up every hard question you hear, and then write or craft a good answer. Practice (or role-play) the answer with a staff person. Practice delivering your answer with confidence until it flows smoothly. This is called scripting. And scripting in its highest form is a tool that will make your job easier and more enjoyable.

Here's an example: I once had an office on the 75th floor of the Columbia Tower, one of the oldest and most iconic buildings in Seattle, which had a problem with the wiring. I called maintenance, and they sent a tech. I noticed that he had a belt full of small and unique tools that I had never seen before. He used three of these to quickly solve my problem. It was slick.

Since his tools were unlike any collection I'd ever seen, I asked him where he found them. "I've made all these myself," he told me. "Every time I'm faced with a new challenge that a better tool will solve, I go make that tool. I keep making, collecting, and discarding a few. Right now, I figure these tools make my job easier, and they're fun to use. It's a hobby of mine." What a great metaphor!

Now, to understand the parallel: chiropractors have the opportunity to tinker with tool making too. Not long ago, I spent time customizing a script (a tool) for a client. She had been having the common trouble of explaining what I call "the money"—the payment options and obligations—on her care plans, and she wanted to polish that up and take care of it for good. She had pulled the framework of what she should say from one of my existing scripts but had a unique concern. And so I modified the tool for her. Then we role-played it back and forth a couple of times, until it was smooth as silk. She went away happy as a lark.

It just took a couple of minutes, and it was a pleasure to do. Hey, making scripting tools is a hobby of mine.

And this doctor now has a whole tool belt full of scripts that make her practice easier and more enjoyable, and at least one tool that makes handling the money a lot easier as well.

28

Success Language

One of the best parts of my job is the front row seat it gives me to life change. I've seen discouraged and defeated doctors, just days away from packing it in, go to incredible heights, loving the journey and process as much as the destination.

It's my job as a coach to find and fan sparks of success into roaring fires. That frequently means assessing where a doctor is, mentally and emotionally, and then laying out a game plan that takes the doctor to their desired goals.

During the game itself, I play three parts: coach, cheerleader, and referee. I call the plays from the sidelines, cheer my clients on as they execute the plays, and make sure they stay "in bounds," which in this case means that they don't get into negative conversations about themselves or run the wrong way when adversity shows up.

Throughout the whole process, I have regular coach, cheerleader, and referee conversations with the player (client). And those conversations have taught me something fascinating. I've noticed that every successful doctor has or develops the same way of communicating. Not only is there a predictable attitude, but the same topics and phrases come up as well.

Winners start off their conversations by talking about their wins. They aren't bragging; they're just excited about their success. Winners who talk about their wins create energy in those conversations. And what do they do with that energy? That's right; they pick another target or goal and set out to win at that too.

Again and again, a predictable six-step conversation emerged. Here are the steps:

1. **Wins:** Even tiny wins are wins, and they're where successful communicators direct their focus. (This also assures that they're in the game and swinging at the ball.)

2. **Near-term goals:** Their previous win produces energy that they carry to the next target, step, or project. Their near-term goals are realistic, require "right now" action, and are no more than six weeks out.

3. **Action steps:** These are the things that a winner is motivated to do and needs to do to reach their near-term goals. There is no success without action. Successful people take action.

4. **Brainstorming:** This is where coach and player put their heads together and strategize.

5. **Problems:** Everyone has them, and winners never expect or pretend to be problem free. However, they don't focus on their problems, and they certainly don't talk about problems at the top of a coaching call. They aren't problem focused—they're solution focused.

6. **Affirmation:** Winners don't end a conversation without a comment about a positive projected fact about the future! My favorites are "It's all an adventure!" and "Kickin' butt and takin' names." I never knew what that second one meant, but I've always liked it.

This formula really works. I had a particularly frightened client who obsessed over her problems, wasn't making much progress, and frankly was no fun to talk to. Then I told her that all of our future calls had to follow the successful pattern that begins with wins, near-term goals, action steps, and brainstorming—then tackles the problems. I sold the process well, and she was up for it.

On our next phone call, though, she dove right into the crisis of the day and started spiraling out of control. "Hey, remember the new protocol?" I asked. She didn't. I reminded her and required eleven minutes of discussion about her recent wins before we talked about anything else.

It went slowly at first, because she wasn't very good at talking about wins. Then, with more confidence, she started listing one positive event after another. Eleven minutes into the conversation, she was a new person—excited and ready to set some new near-term goals. "My problems don't seem so bad. I guess I'm really headed in the right direction."

Wow! This was coaching dynamite!

Teaching a struggling person how to talk like a winner makes my coaching calls into what amounts to a foreign language lesson. Like learning a foreign language, permanent change doesn't happen overnight or without resistance. Old habits die hard, but results are amazing. It wasn't long before that particular client noticed when she got off target or backslid into a bad habit and had the ability to self-correct. She liked the new her a lot more, and so did I.

By the way, she also added 120-plus visits a week to her practice.

In summary, winners (successful people) have similar thought patterns that show up in their speech. Those patterns are either innate or acquired. If you teach yourself to communicate like a winner, success can quickly follow. But remember, if you don't act differently, you'll get the same results you always have.

Warning: Steer clear of the pessimists who eagerly relay the next impending disaster. Instead, support the new you by hanging out with people who speak success fluently and demand the same of you. Find groups that share great action-oriented information, set goals, share their wins, and engage in a little friendly competition.

Here's to your success!

29

What I Learned from Oprah

I happened to be watching TV one day when Oprah Winfrey had a group of very heavy women on her program. The subject was the heartbreak that comes when diets don't work.

Each of the women had lost more than one hundred pounds, only to gain at least that much back again. They didn't want to gain the weight back, of course, but none of them had been able to avoid it. They described it as a mystery and lamented that they were powerless to stop it. No one was happy—including Oprah.

Statistics show that Oprah's guests aren't the only people in that spot. Numerous studies show that when people lose that much weight, they frequently gain it back again.

However, in the tearful descriptions of their roller-coaster weight loss and uncontrollable gain, I noticed that each person clearly but unconsciously explained her mistake, and yet not one person mentioned it, including Oprah.

Each of the women got off their diet.

Each person explained something to the effect of "I lost the weight and quit going to the support group meetings." Or "I stopped being so strict about food." Or "I quit checking in with my counselor and quit getting weighed every day."

In short, what I saw was that this was a group of people who had something that was naturally hard for them to do without help (eat right and exercise), which they'd then handled beautifully using systems, rules, and external motivation.

But here's the insanity: after all this help worked, they dropped their programs like hot potatoes (without the sour cream, bacon, and chives), even though every weight loss program triples in effectiveness when the participant checks in with a coach.

Here's my question: Why didn't one—and I mean just one— person on that stage say, "I know that I'll need systems, rules, and external motivation the rest of my life. Staying in my skinny jeans (or whatever their motivation) is worth it to me. I'll NEVER quit my program!"

But this isn't a chapter about weight loss. Have you ever heard this one?

"I used to spend marketing time to get new patients, but I quit."

"Why did you quit?"

"Because it worked."

That's just as crazy.

Even crazier is this: Every year I speak to doctors desperate to grow their practices. Invariably, their best-ever years in practice were the ones where they worked with this or that practice coach.

"Why did you quit?" I ask.

It's always the same response. "I learned everything that coach could teach me."

In other words, because it worked.

They're missing the point. Let's go back to the weight loss parallel. Is there anyone who doesn't know that eating less and exercising more will make you lose weight? Yet when it comes to success in anything, it isn't what you *know*—it's what you *do with what you know*. And the fact is that you do your best work when you use successful systems, rules, and external motivation like seminars, coaching calls, and networking with special interest groups.

The simple knowledge that someone is going to check in with you about your practice, help you process new information, and offer a better perspective and encouragement helps you focus on success.

Don't make friends with mediocrity. Hire the right coach, and then do everything they say with all your intensity and passion. Unlike the dieters on TV, stay in the system, do the program, and stay in touch with your coach, even after you discover success.

Because once you succeed, you can look for the next level of success and then the next and the next.

I gained thirty pounds right after I got married. I found out how much I gained using a talking scale in a crowded store. How stupid was that?

I kicked the button on the scale as we were walking by and heard a robotic voice say, "Get on the scale. Get on the scale." So I obediently stepped on, only to hear, "Hey, you guys, one at a time!"

No, I didn't hear that, but I think it's funny. What I did hear was a number that was my high school weight plus thirty pounds.

I looked at my wife in horror. She was laughing. In a matter of days, I was sitting with a counselor in a commercial weight-loss program, learning everything I could about how to lose weight. I love systems and formulas, and I was back to my high school weight in a few short months, and then I stepped into maintenance.

That was more than twenty-five years ago, and I still check in with that group from time to time, just to keep in touch.

Best advice? Get coached. Stay coached.

30

How to Pick a Coach for Your Practice

A friend of mine is an Ironman triathlete. He has four different coaches for this event: one for biking, one for running, and two for swimming. I asked him if all that was necessary, and he gave me the best answer I could think of.

"All the guys who are hitting the times I want to hit have at least three coaches. I've improved by 20 percent in each area since I've been coached, and I'm not in this thing alone."

There really isn't any question in athletics about the value of coaches. All serious athletes hire coaches. Period. So why is there any controversy in chiropractic about using coaches or consultants? I've met plenty of good doctors who were stuck at a fraction of their potential just because they couldn't or wouldn't get some help. Their reasons for putting up with years of disappointment and mediocrity are varied, but most often translate into "I just didn't know who to trust."

By contrast, many doctors have become experts at using practice coaches. When asked why, their answers are roughly the same as the athletes.

"Most successful doctors I know use or have used coaches. I'm helping more people, having more fun, and making more money than ever before. And I'm not in this thing alone."

Do coaches cost you money or make you money? I teach clients to compute their return on investment (ROI) from the fees they spend on consulting. A low ROI for my clients is an eleven to one return. That begs the question: If you could double or triple your practice, cut the stress in half (which will double your fun), and get eleven dollars in exchange for every dollar spent in the process, wouldn't you try? Of course you would, but how do you choose a practice coach who's right for you?

For the doctor who's ready to make a change and wants to choose the best practice coach for them, I have a short list of things to look for in a coach or consultant.

1. Choose a coach who is doing what you want to do.

Today's market is different than it was five years ago. If a coach doesn't have their own clinics and isn't doing well in today's market, you may be left with systems and programs that are outdated, or worse, just don't work. If you are looking for help attracting new patients, how does the coach do with marketing their own offices? If you want to develop associates, does your coach know how?

2. Don't settle for being just one of the herd.

Big shows in big rooms with lots of people and inspirational music may be entertaining, but who's looking out for you personally? If you're passed off to a junior employee (sometimes not even a chiropractor) instead of being known and guided by one of the principle teachers, that could be a problem. Think of it like this:

Do you want your children in a classroom with 166 other students, or sixteen?

3. Get specific answers to specific problems.

Some consultants say they'll work on your headspace, and you'll figure out the rest. How does that work? If you need new patients, you need specific, step-by-step procedures that you can copy in your practice in order to produce new patients. Some groups seem to miss the point of systems. There's a right and wrong way to do everything in and out of the office, so find a group that has tested and polished the "right way" solutions to your problems so you don't have to reinvent the wheel. Isn't that what you're paying them for?

4. Insist on the Golden Rule.

Some doctors have come to me with questions about the ethics of certain groups. Here's my answer: If a group teaches you to do a hard sell instead of educate and lead patients, that's a red flag. If you would have any hesitation about sending your friends and family to a doctor using that group's systems, they aren't for you. Remember, if you're going to love your practice as long as you're in it, you need to treat patients with love and respect and "do unto others as you would have them do unto you."

5. Insist on good value.

Price out your coaching options; with some groups, the fees are huge. Others are so low you wonder how they can provide the service they promise—the answer is that frequently they can't.

I'm also not comfortable with paying a percentage of your practice's income increase as a fee. In my view, that punishes you for your success. I like knowing what things will cost up front. Instead, run the math. See how much it will cost to learn and implement a solid, proven program, and then work your tail off to increase your ROI and make it a great bargain.

6. Look for a personal resonance with the leader and group.

The principle consultant's message should click in your head, heart, and gut. You should look forward to being coached by that person and embrace their mission. Surround yourself with people who are in it to help people, have fun, and be successful. Then do it yourself in that same order.

7. Get a coach when you're ready, and give it everything you've got.

Being the right client is as important as finding the right coach. Decide that you'll be the best client that your coach ever had, and determine to be the client that hears his coach say, "You're kidding? You did all that already?"

31

My New Coaching Coach

I have mixed feelings about telling you about my experience as a person being coached, rather than doing the coaching, but I learned a ton. Most chiropractic practice consultants don't get to sit in another coach's classes. We spend so much time on our own seminars and coaching schedule that it's rare to find the time to sharpen our skills.

But what's really important here is that not only am I learning good things, I have also found it's interesting (and instructive) to pay attention to how I'm approaching the challenge of getting the most out of the material I'm paying for.

I decided at the beginning I'd be the dream client I hope for and would hold myself responsible for getting the most I can out of my time in the group. Here are the thirteen things I do to make that happen. I call them:

A Baker's Dozen Tips for Getting the Most Out of Your Coach

1. I'm responsible, and it's up to me to get as much as I can out of the whole coaching experience.

2. I make quick use of the material to stay motivated and excited. It's up to me to do that.

3. I study the material between 36 and 120 minutes a day, five to six days a week.

   How do I know about the time so precisely? I work out every day except Sundays, including thirty-six minutes of cardio training on a StairMaster. During that time, I watch and listen to recorded webinars or streamed MP3 files. When I hear a great idea, I email those thoughts to myself and my assistant from my iPhone.)

4. My assistant prints the "great idea" emails and three-hole punches them for my notebook.

5. I transcribe parts or all of more pertinent webinars. I read and reread those notes.

6. I head into the office early to be alone and review my notes.

7. I attend all of my coach's workshops and show up with tons of written questions.

8. I send my coach super-short emails, with one or two questions maximum to make it easier for my coach to answer.

9. I make every effort to be online for live webinar training, and I contribute to the conversation.

10. I share what I'm learning with my assistant. When I can, I pull my CA into my office for the webinar trainings, and we learn together. Remember, "the teacher always learns more than the pupil," and I want to absorb what I'm learning—so I teach.

11. I jump in and start using new material ASAP, with notes in hand if needed, and push to make changes and improvements. At sixty-five, I'm officially the old dog with the new trick.

12. I'm careful to do exactly what I'm asked to do, exactly the way I'm asked to do it, and I never disagree.

13. I race with other people in the program to make it more fun to implement new stuff.

If *you're* willing to do this for your consultant or coach, you'll make them look like a genius. By the way, that's my goal with my coach.

32

Not Knowing What You Don't Know

Think about it—that's a scary situation.

If you don't know what you don't know, great peril could be just around the corner. Or you could be missing buried treasure just by an inch, for decades.

I can't tell you the number of times I've seen a DC shake their head and offer the now all-too-common lament: "If I'd only known this years ago."

On occasion, I've even helped doctors run the math on their disasters, actually calculating what I've come to call the "ignorance tax."

One small tweak to an ROF script can lead to an increase of thousands of return visits a year. "Damn. Not knowing that was sure expensive. What else don't I know?"

But it's not your fault. If you don't know what you don't know, you think everyone has a devil of a time getting this or that done. You don't know that there's a better, faster, easier, or cheaper way.

But what if you're just one number off on a winning ticket that pays out in increased patient compliance; a bigger, lower-stress practice; and literally a million-dollar increase when calculated over years?

Okay, how do I do that?

Get connected. Get in the stream of new information and best practices.

Okay, get connected, but to whom? You?

Maybe, but let's talk about what to look for in a more general sense. Here's how to learn what you don't know:

1. Ask your DC friends who are working with a coaching or management group. If one of your buddies likes their coach, see if there's an introductory offer for an upcoming event.

2. When you're at the event, see if there's a free consultation available with one of the coaches in the group. Bring a ton of questions, and make sure you tell them what you're doing. Ask for feedback.

3. Pick out three to five of the group's best and brightest clients to speak to during breaks. Ask them about their practices, how they like the consulting company, and what they've learned.

4. Ask yourself if you like the feel of the group and if the approach fits your personality.

5. Run the math: If you joined this group for a year, would you be better off than if you didn't? You want to at least make a five-to-one ROI on your money, preferably ten-to-one.

6. If they have a seminar special, join in and keep the momentum going.

7. Get a full practice evaluation, complete with personalized recommendations, and then do them.

Hey, this isn't rocket science. If the sharp people in the group are doing well, decide that you will learn what they know and do at least as well as they do.

This is better than finding out you could have had a better practice and better life just because of what you didn't know.

33

Real Power

Where does the real power to transform your practice actually come from?

My golf instructor was showing me a video clip of what he called the perfect drive. "Everything is all lined up and headed in the same direction, and each piece accelerates the next until maximum power and speed are reached right at impact." He was gushing now. "When you hit the ball that way, you barely feel it, and it goes like a rocket!"

Sometime later, I hit the ball exactly that way, and he was right; it felt effortless.

That shot has a lot to teach us chiropractors about how to create real power and passion to transform our practices. Let me explain.

I've known and coached some of the most successful chiropractors in the country. I've helped brand-new graduates grow by hundreds of visits a week and become super-successful. I've guided already successful doctors to replicate their talents in associates and build and sell satellite offices.

In each case, the power came from the same place as a good golf swing: the right essentials, all lined up and heading in the right direction.

When you think about it, that's exceptionally good news. It means there's a formula or a recipe. And if there's a recipe, you can "whip up a batch" of the same success and power —if you're willing to follow the same steps.

I've been working with practices that succeed for a long time, and I'm sure I understand the right steps and the right sequence. Here they are:

First, you must have a strong VISION.

Every successful chiropractor sees themselves as successful, and the more successful they are, the clearer that vision is. We've talked about the importance of vision in several earlier chapters, but it's important to mention here, too. With a clear vision, your subconscious mind is constantly seeking opportunity, solving problems, and moving you forward as if drawn by an invisible force.

Second, you need GOALS.

The energy created by a strong vision must be given a task. That's what your goals are—the work it will take to fulfill your vision.

Set goals that are just out of your reach. They must challenge you.

Make goals clear and defined. They should never confuse you.

Review these goals every day. You must never forget them.

Third, you need some ACTION.

Do you understand how a strong vision and clear goals create spontaneous energy and action? Think back to when you were in high school, and your girlfriend or boyfriend was at a friend's house. I remember the night I hitchhiked eighty miles and arrived at three o'clock in the morning, just as energetic as can be. Seeing my girlfriend was my vision, and I had a goal.

With a strong vision, clear goals, and the right action steps, things start to happen almost automatically. You see what you want in your vision and define it with your goals, and then your subconscious mind sends you on the mission of building the practice of your dreams with your action steps.

I've got some more great news here. **Everything you need to do to be successful, someone else has already done.** Isn't that exciting? First, it means it can be done, and second (and this is the best part) there's a path to follow.

Here's what super-successful chiropractors do: They keep their ears open for what's really working, and then they search like crazy for the best action steps to fulfill their vision and reach their goals. They follow those steps to the letter.

If you're smart, you'll do the same.

Okay, we have a vision, goals, and action steps, and here's where real power comes from: **they must be in alignment.**

No one should understand this point better than chiropractors. When your vision is off to one side and your goals are stuck out to the other, you cut off the life flow and lose power. So please take my advice—do everything needed to get back in alignment! That's where real power is.

Fourth, your conversation must be positive, encouraging, and clear of any "victim-speak."

You know what I mean. There can be no "why me, poor me" comments, or you're dead in the water. The most accurate predictor of failure, as far as I have observed, is "victim-speak." Avoid it, and those who speak it, like the plague.

Fifth, you must make a commitment.

Here's where good old-fashioned determination fits in. The wisest people throughout history all know that the person who refuses to quit is the one who has the best chance of winning.

Now put the pieces together. With a strong vision, clear goals, proven formulas and recipes, positive self-talk, and commitment, you have everything lined up and headed in the same direction. It's like my golf coach's video clip; it's the perfect drive that produces the real power to build and transform your practice.

34

Eliminate Stress in Your Practice

Dr. Dave loves chiropractic, has a great personal chiropractic story, and used to love going to the office. But recently he told a colleague, only half joking, "I love chiropractic. It's the practice I hate."

I asked him why he felt that way. "It's too stressful," he answered.

Stress can put a knot in your stomach and a frown on your face and leave you exhausted and sick.

For too many chiropractors, their practice is a major source of stress. What was once a delight becomes a source of mental anguish.

Stress can pile up quickly and take away the enjoyment of your practice. Instead of looking forward to taking care of people, you slog through another day, another year, just seconds from yet another heavy sigh, secretly counting down the time to retirement.

The good news is it doesn't have to be that way.

You can eliminate the stress in your practice and enjoy being a chiropractor again, all while helping more people, having more fun, and making more money.

The following are the five most common practice stresses that can leave you grinding your teeth at night. I'll give you solid, practical strategies and solutions to get rid of each stress and love your practice again.

Stressor #1: You do not have enough new patients.

Not bringing in enough new patients will produce a host of problems, including a feeling of failed purpose, small practice volume, low energy, and poor collections. The lack of new patients is the single biggest practice stressor for most chiropractors by a factor of ten to one.

Solution: I've helped literally thousands of doctors beat this problem. The solution is simple, and results can be dramatic. First, quit complaining about the need to market chiropractic and yourself, and just get good at it. Every business needs to market, and the medical profession has a $1 trillion industry shilling for it. We don't, so just embrace the opportunity and do it.

Start by hanging a marketing calendar in your back office. Then fill it up with three internal and three external new patient programs. Spend between three and seven hours a week telling the chiropractic story and offering help.

Hot Tip: Learn how to manage a marketing CA who goes into the community to do screenings, corporate health fairs, and massage events. The marketing CA brings in new patients while you stay in the office taking care of established patients. Never be without one of these. This is the most logical next hire in all of chiropractic.

Stressor #2: Your team doesn't perform to your standards.

Your day starts off stressfully if your staff arrives late and poorly dressed and won't take care of you or your patients the way you'd like. This stress distracts you from patient care because you know the phone work, patient scheduling, billing, etc., are in bad repair.

It seems like no matter what you do, you can't get the performance you're looking for from your team. The growing frustration invites the daily thought, "I can hardly wait to get out of here!"

Solution: For just a moment, think of your practice as a half-time show at a college football game; you and your staff are the marching band. You want your performance to be precise and energetic and impress the fans. How will it get that way? For major colleges, the process starts months before football season begins. The band takes to the field late at night in an empty stadium to practice each and every song, all the dance moves, and every formation—again and again and again.

You need a team that works with that kind of precision, anticipating your needs and caring for your patients like honored guests. The key is practice. Train your standards on every aspect of office management—from how to answer the phone to Days One and Two procedures—and how to handle every possible situation. And then practice them again and again and again.

Hot Tip: Tell your staff, "Next Tuesday, we're running through the New Patient Day One routine from start to finish. I want everyone to have the scripts memorized. Amy will play the part of the new patient. Here are the scripts. Any questions?" Consistent training over time is the key here.

Stressor #3: You have an office full of demanding, spoiled, ungrateful patients.

Some patients are so demanding that you end up in debates over whether you're adjusting them right. "Don't think you got it, Doc. Try again." Or "I want you to do this one free. The last one didn't work." If this is happening to you, the fact is you created the problem by allowing the behavior, and you can also fix it.

Solution: Right at the start, you need to frame the relationship. A positive statement that installs you as the leader and the patient as the follower, and explaining it in a way where they happily agree is essential.

My script for new patients starts this way: "Before we get started, let me tell you how we do things..." This announces that the doctor has a proven, trusted process. Then take control by doing a strong Day One and Day Two, explaining the best path to their goal of wellness. Extract their commitments to your way of doing things.

Be authoritative. Patients respect you when they're convinced you know what you're doing. If they don't respect you, maybe they're in the wrong office.

Hot Tip: If you've never "fired" a patient before, try it. It's an empowering feeling. Your staff will probably thank you, and everyone feels better. Ask your CAs who's the worst patient, and find that patient another DC.

Stressor #4: You have a case of too much month and not enough money.

Another way to put that is—you have poor collections.

Granted, most low-cash stress goes away when you market and start bringing in more patients. But I've seen busy, successful practices leave over $100,000 a year rotting in the Accounts Receivable office and later write most of it off as bad debt. That hard-earned cash could have gone home with you.

Solution: Set a goal to collect 96 percent of AR after your managed care organization (MCO) write-offs.

First, standardize all patient payment plans, giving them four options: prepay, use health-care financing (like CareCredit), auto-debit directly from a bank account, and pay as you go. That will fix the money going into AR.

Now for getting the money out that's already in AR: Each week meet with your CA over a fresh paper copy of an aged AR. Identify the twelve most troubled accounts, starting with those carrying large balances, bad payment histories, and poor security. Then make specific assignments to the staff to audit, rebill, call the insurance company, call the patient, call the attorney (for personal injury cases), or send a collection letter.

Hot Tip: Require a sixty-second daily check-in from the biller on the assigned work. When two or three accounts resolve, add two or three more. Schedule weekly AR meetings and repeat the process.

In no time, you'll be hard-pressed to find twelve troubled accounts, and you'll put tons of extra cash in your pocket.

Stressor #5: You're the prisoner of your own success.

You have a busy practice, wonderful patients, delightful staff, and a great income. But your dirty little secret is that you're working at close to capacity, and you can't take time away without damaging (even crashing) the practice. Two weeks off could cost tens of thousands of dollars.

Solution: Would you like to have four to six weeks off a year while the practice purrs like a kitten in your absence?

Hire an associate with compatible goals and formulate a well-laid-out plan for a win-win relationship. Lead and manage your associate based on replicating your success in them.

Hot Tip: When the associate is fully trained, let them handle the practice solo on a Friday. Check their performance and make corrections. Sometime later, ask them to cover for your four-day weekend. Eventually, you'll be ready to take a full week off, and then do that several times a year.

If you want to love both chiropractic and your practice for a lifetime, identify the stressors and deal with them head on—the earlier, the better.

35

The Quick Fix

Sorry to break it to you, but I think you already know that the "quick fix" is neither quick nor a fix. Look around you. What do they call the quick-fix dieter? Plump. What do they call the quick-fix exerciser? Out of shape. What do they call the doctor who's looking for the quick-fix for a struggling practice? Unsuccessful.

As a group, we humans are pretty smart. We put a man on the moon and all that. And in our heart of hearts, we know that quick fixes really don't work. However, every year, horrific golfers (whose equipment already surpasses their ability) spend tens of millions of dollars on brand-new clubs, looking for a quick fix—and then they continue to play terrible golf. It defines insanity.

If I told you about some of the equally pathetic schemes some doctors have sunk thousands of dollars into, you'd be shaking your head in no time.

If there's a Hall of Shame (dumb things that cost a lot and don't ever work), is there a Hall of Fame (smart things that give great value and success while reducing stress)? Yes.

But here are the bigger questions: Why should you trust me to tell you? How can you know what I say will work?

Great questions! I'll give you the one test that *never* lies. It's worth a million dollars. I'll give it to you for free, but you'll have to dig it out.

Here we go.

Interview five people who lost more than fifty pounds and kept it off. Ask them how they did it. Then interview five people who were out of shape then got fit and stayed fit. Now interview five people who actually dropped their golf score by twenty strokes and now consistently shoot in the high seventies and low eighties.

Then interview a chiropractor who used to struggle terribly but now sees an extra one to two hundred visits a week, and yet works half as hard. They will all tell the same story. Not one of them will tell you it was a quick fix.

Since what you'll find is the ONLY WAY that really works, shouldn't we already be listening?

(By the way, I know that ALL CAPS is the writing equivalent of yelling. You would yell, too, if you regularly spoke to nice doctors who do the wrong thing again and again, for decades, expecting a different result.)

So what *does* work every time?

I know DCs who consistently produce more than fifty new patients a month. They're never looking for a quick fix. I know golfers with a +5 handicap. They frequently play with clubs they've had for years. The thin and fit—and I mean those who used to be really out of shape and have lost quite a bit of weight—all do the same things.

They commit to a proven plan, use expert and peer support, and stick to it.

The dieter, exerciser, and golfer each use a proven system, enlist a coach, and surround themselves with friends who support them.

They know that any plateau or setback can be solved with a system, support, and stick-to-itiveness.

What does that look like for the chiropractor?

First, join a management company. Is it self-serving for me to say this? Of course it is, but that doesn't make it untrue. Face it, if you haven't found the answers by yourself by now, you aren't going to. The best way to choose a consultant is the same way most people choose a chiropractor—ask your friends and neighbors. Most groups pay for themselves ten or twenty times over. This won't cost you, it'll pay you.

Next, assemble your own mastermind group to challenge and encourage you. Most of the time you can find people in your management group who are eager to cheer you on and give you a push when you need it. I encourage my clients to clump up in groups of five or six and push each other.

Last, set aside two hours a week to work *on* your practice, not *in* the practice. Working *on* the practice is like detailing an abused or neglected car—your interest in and enjoyment of that car goes up as you invest yourself in the details.

Does it take work? Of course it does, but I know many doctors who now have millions in the bank because of that single principle. Don't know how or what needs work first? That's a good reason to hire a coach who can help you with systems and spend time with friends headed in the same direction you want to go.

Since chiropractors work with the power that created the universe, why are we so slow to learn the truths that continue to rule the universe? Tell me, does anyone (and I mean anyone) think you'll get washboard abs from the ab gimmicks you see on TV?

36

What I Learned from Golf

You know the old joke, "Why do they call it golf? Because %&#@ and &@!% (two other popular four-letter words) were already taken."

Recently, I've run into a number of doctors who are using far too many four-letter words to describe not only their golf game but also their chiropractic practices. And, not so surprisingly, for very similar reasons.

Their good days on the links and in the office are mainly accidents, while most days produce only disappointment and frustration. After playing golf and practicing chiropractic for decades, they're still struggling terribly with both.

During a recent golf game, my doctor friend turned to me after hitting two balls into the lake and said, "The only thing I hate more than this game is my practice." Ouch.

Let me clear up a couple of points. No, he wasn't one of my consulting clients, and he didn't hate chiropractic—just chiropractic *practice*.

On the other hand, I know some excellent golfers with single-digit handicaps, and I know a number of very successful DCs with big practices, low stress, lots of money, and tons of free time.

Here's the not-so-surprising connection:

Great golfers and successful chiropractors have an amazing amount in common.

In fact, the success checklists for both golf and chiropractic are interchangeable.

Let's take a brief look at what golf has to teach us about succeeding in chiropractic practice.

1. Don't be tricked into the "quick fix" or "magic wand" mentality.

Ever read the cover of *Golf* magazine?

"Smash It Down the Center EVERY TIME!"

"NEVER Three-Putt Again!"

The ads on the inside cover are even worse, with promises of perfect clubs that will never fail you. Never mind that you've bought a brand-new set every year for as long as you can remember and still don't play any better. Just get this new set with "NEW Secret Technology!"

In chiropractic, when someone promises that this software or that device will bring an instant end to every challenge you face, you can plan on a disappointing result. I know doctors with storage units full of years of expensive fads or gimmick purchases that guaranteed they'd produce success "Just Like Magic!"

Real change in both golf and chiropractic takes time and practice, but thankfully, less of both than you might think. Anyway, if a good golfer can beat you with the clubs you threw away eight years ago, maybe it's not the clubs.

2. Get help.

Every professional golfer (and they make the most money) has a coach. All of them pay experts to watch, advise, and cheer them on. One of my favorite facts about top performers in every field is that they *all* have coaches. The highly successful—and this is no small point—learn to act on their coach's advice. They work at being teachable.

In chiropractic, the *most* successful DCs have coaches. Find a coach who has helped people who are like you and who do what you want to do, then do exactly what your coach tells you. It doesn't make sense to not listen, right?

Speaking of advice, I'm willing to bet your golf coach sent you to the practice tee right after correcting your slice, right? That's my next point.

3. Practice.

Every top golfer practices before and/or after their game. Without exception, great golfers practice dozens of hours for every hour of tournament play.

When I attended the US Open Championship one year near Seattle, I was impressed by the hours the best in the world still spent on the practice tee, in the sand trap, and on the putting green.

If you could use a little improvement *and* are motivated, here's a list of procedures in your practice that you should practice:
- Converting new patient prospects to treating patients
- Getting patients to commit to and stay in good care plans
- Explaining and getting commitment on financial plans
- Handling the patient who wants to quit a good care plan
- Converting a patient from relief, correction, and strengthening to wellness

- Both successful golfers and chiropractors are always working on some part of their game. I've been at it for more than forty years, and I still need the practice.

By the way, a correct golf swing or practice script can feel uncomfortable at first. That's why you practice—to work out the rough spots.

Sound like a lot of work? I think struggling in a failing practice, just barely making it each month, is a lot harder. Let's learn from great golfers so we can help a ton of people, have a gob of fun, and be more successful.

37

Flawless Delegation

Dr. Smith was having another bad day. He was running behind again and felt out of control, which left him so distracted that his patients could sense it. What's worse, it was only 10:30 a.m. on Monday.

For the umpteenth time, he asked himself, "Why does practice have to be so hard?"

His desk and pockets were littered with small scraps of paper with scribbled reminders of important tasks, but he was losing that battle. "There's just too much to do," he said under his breath.

A recent new patient program had caused the practice to grow, which was good for the bottom line, but his stress had also increased exponentially. Sadly, experience taught him that whenever the practice grew like this, he'd lose control of the details, the pressure would build, and the growth would slip away.

"Why even bother trying to build the practice?"

Dr. Smith worried about all the loose ends and uncompleted tasks at the office while he was home, and his stress stole the joy from his time with his family.

As if this wasn't bad enough, he also worried about his family while taking care of patients.

At the end of this day, he slumped into his desk chair, completely exhausted, wondering how he could finish the month, let alone keep this up until retirement. There had to be a better way.

Across town, Dr. Jones had just finished another busy, exciting day in the clinic. He loved the way the whole team pulled together, with everyone doing their special piece to produce yet another stellar performance that was more fun than work.

"Here are your stats, Doctor. I think you're going to like 'em." His CA handed him the day's numbers neatly written on a Post-it note.

After a quick review, he smiled and looked up to say, "Great work, team. We rock!"

So why does Dr. Smith feel like he's carrying the weight of the world on his shoulders, and Dr. Jones feels like his much larger practice is a game?

And why does Dr. Smith do three times the work and yet see a fraction of the patients Dr. Jones does?

Years ago, Dr. Jones had a similar struggle, but he learned a simple step-by-step process for delegation, and that process empowered his team and cut his workload to a fraction.

Dr. Smith had also tried delegating, but, according to him, it blew up on him—several times. After discovering serious staff errors, he was left muttering, "If you want something done right, you have to do it yourself."

Dr. Jones, on the other hand, did only what he was required to do and delegated everything else. He knew for certain that each delegated task was being done exactly like he designed it. This knowledge alone allowed him to be "in the moment" at the clinic with patients, and also at home with his family.

Two caring chiropractors. Two entirely different experiences. One was buried by an avalanche of poorly done or uncompleted tasks. The other was hard-pressed to even call his practice work.

As fate would have it, Smith and Jones—who'd never met before—ended up at the same seminar and in the coffee line together.

Dr. Smith read Dr. Jones's name tag and said, "Heard you see lots of people. You must work your tail off."

"We're busy, but it's pretty low stress. I cut my workload to almost nothing several years ago when I started to delegate. Most days it runs as smooth as silk," replied Jones.

"I tried delegating, and it was a disaster." Smith grimaced as he shook his head.

"My first attempts at delegating were pretty bad, too, but I learned a simple process that works like a charm. Want me to diagram it out for you?"

"Won't let you outta here until you do." Both men smiled.

The two new friends grabbed a table, and Dr. Jones proceeded to teach what he called the "Seven Secrets to Flawless Delegation."

1. You have no right to expect anything that isn't written down. This assumption requires you to list everything you want, which clears up most misunderstandings and synchronizes expectations. Hold yourself to this axiom, and you'll have a better life.

   Hot Tip: Each task on a written checklist is delegable, and every position has a checklist.

2. Write each delegated task out step-by-step, exactly as you want it done. Draw up a flow chart, attach a script, or copy a page from your practice management manual—just make sure it's crystal clear.

   Hot Tip: Every position should have a delegated-task book.

3. Discuss how the delegated tasks serve the clinic goals. This is the big WHY. The task makes sense to you, the doctor who needs to delegate, but you still need to put it into context for your staff, relating it back to your philosophy, clinic vision, purpose, and mission.
   Hot Tip: Connect each delegated task back to a higher purpose.

4. Demonstrate the task for the staff. Most of us learn by watching and copying what we see, so give staff a good model to follow.
   Hot Tip: Record videos of tasks being done right, and share them with the trainee.

5. Make sure your staff can explain the what, where, when, why, who, and how of the task. Ask questions to test their understanding of the delegated task.
   Hot Tip: Start with simple questions about task mechanics, and expand to more complex applications.

6. Work with the staff until they can demonstrate the delegated task to the standard. This is the only way that you know they can do what you're delegating.
   Hot Tip: Each task should require an official sign-off before it's considered delegated.

7. Perform regular inspections. Don't micromanage, but regularly inspect delegated tasks to make sure they're being handled appropriately. Ask questions, give feedback, and fine-tune the training process. This step is the key to strong delegation and to keeping the task in good repair.
   Hot Tip: Remember, you get what you inspect, not what you expect.

"Ouch," Smith lamented when Jones was done. "This is too much. I'm already buried. I wouldn't even know where I'd start."

Jones smiled. "I know just how you feel. I felt that way myself, but I found delegating was the only way out of my mess. And it saved a lot more time than it took."

Jones explained that he picked a few simple tasks first, used the seven-step process, and got three projects delegated and functioning well.

"Both my CA and I were so pleased that we were motivated to do more. That's how I built my delegating skills. I just kept tackling the next task. It's how I've now delegated 80 percent of my work," Jones told Smith. "And there's a side benefit I haven't even mentioned. This year, I'll take a full six weeks off with the family, and I'll still have my best-ever year financially."

"What? Really? How?"

"Using the seven-step delegation process over time has my associates and CAs running on rails. I leave for a great vacation, but the delegated tasks stay in place. Everything functions beautifully."

Dr. Smith just stared at the seven-point outline Jones had sketched. It actually made sense. In that instant, he decided to change. What did he have to lose?

Fast-forward two weeks. Dr. Smith is proud he's already delegated four tasks, and his CA appreciates the clarity of the seven-step process. He sends Dr. Jones this email:

Subject: 4 tasks delegated, 22 to go!

Hey, Dr. J,

Can't thank you enough. Love the Seven Secrets to Flawless Delegation.

I'm not flawless yet, but I can see the light at the end of the tunnel.

Practice is fun again.

Best,

Dr. S

38

Cutting Back

"Your interview is here, Dr. Lloyd."

I thanked Debbie and finished making a note on my list. I had been advertising for a new associate after building and selling three clinics to associates that year. I could see the candidate through my office window that looks into the hallway. A well-dressed young man with an expensive haircut sat in the waiting area, looking totally relaxed.

I walked to my office door, greeted him, and took two steps forward to shake his hand as he stood. "Nice to meet you. Come on in and have a seat."

I like developing chiropractors and enjoy the process of meeting and discerning who the right candidate is. I've spent so much time learning what I need to do to be successful, not to mention learning what *not* to do, that it's satisfying and rewarding to take a new doctor on the right path, seeing someone else's dreams and potential become reality. However, it has to be the right doctor.

In the first few moments of an interview, I watch and listen for interpersonal skills and confidence. I look for posture, eye contact, facial expression—all the things that constitute nonverbal communication. I'm taking the long view from the beginning. I want to be able to see that what I know will translate into success.

First impressions are important and frequently correct. I like confidence, but a little nervousness isn't bad. In order to learn what I have to teach, an associate not only needs to want to learn, but they need to respect *me*, as well as what I teach. I'm watching to see if they have learned for themselves to give respect.

I've also learned to not chase an applicant who puts me in a no-lose situation. My own attitude is completely relaxed.

I noticed that the applicant was wearing a silk shirt and light sweater and too many pastels—not the expected doctor attire of a shirt and tie.

I thought, *He's dressed more expensively than I am... but he's not dressed appropriately.*

As he sat down across the desk from me, I also noticed that he was *too* relaxed. He not only wasn't nervous, he had no respect for my process—maybe no respect for me.

We exchanged pleasantries, and I asked him why he became a chiropractor. I always do this, and I listen for commitment, passion, and excitement. His measured and careful response had none of that.

Just four minutes into the interview, I asked, "What do you want to be doing five years from now?" This is a key question for me. If what he wants to do is what I know how to help him do, maybe we should work together.

I'd given him a chance to paint a gorgeous picture of an exciting future—something I can commit myself to as well. This, above all other questions, produces my best assessment on whether to hire or not.

"I want to be cutting back a little," he said. I knew what he meant, but I was still stunned and needed to make sure I hadn't misinterpreted what he was saying. Sadly, I was right. He repeated himself. *He wanted to cut back.*

He wasn't even in the door, and he was already looking for the exit.

He hadn't even said "I do," and he was thinking about a trial separation.

He said that to the wrong man. I had decided to be a chiropractor when I was eleven years old, and I gave it everything I had for decades. I had my heart broken when a career-ending injury sidelined me from active practice—my highest calling—and he *wanted to cut back.*

In an instant, I knew the right thing to do. "Come with me," I said and stood. He looked surprised and asked where we were going. "I want to show you something," I told him.

In five seconds, we were standing in front of what I wanted to show him—the door. My conviction grew with every step. I pushed the door open, and we both walked outside into the summer sun. I stopped and turned to face him as the door closed behind us. He looked a little confused, but I would fix that.

"I made a decision to become a chiropractor when I was eleven, and I've been practicing for twenty-eight years. Not even once have I ever thought about *cutting back.* I love chiropractic more today than I ever have and don't ever want to cut back or work with anyone who does. This interview is over."

During my short speech, I noticed a gold-badged, top-end Lexus with an older couple sitting in the front and a young, attractive woman âĂŞ probably a girlfriend âĂŞ in the back. I put myself in that father's position. He did not get that car and all the money it took to spoil his son by cutting back.

I imagined that his dad probably knew that Junior took too many things for granted, and all that he had been given didn't have the effect his father had hoped for. "Tell your dad what I told you," I said as I walked back into the office.

Let's you and I make an agreement to never cut back.

Part Three

Make More Money

Taking Care of Your Staff

39

How to Build the Perfect Team

Wow, a PERFECT team? That's a lot of pressure. But let's jump in, break it down, and see how we do.

First, who's the perfect team member? In my view, the perfect team member shows up early, with a great attitude, anticipates the needs of their doctors and patients, and consistently does great work.

What more could you ask for?

Second, what's a perfect team? Doesn't it stand to reason that it's a group of perfect team members functioning in harmony? Sure it does, but what would that look like? For me, it's simple: a clinic that produces high-volume weeks consistently, without a hitch, providing happy patients with great chiropractic care offered by DCs and CAs who are grateful to be a part of the perfect team. Oh, and don't forget, there's a large profit margin.

But can we, in this life, ever get a perfect team? I say yes, but it might look different than you think.

I have to start with a confession. I'm not perfect. In fact, I'm far from it. (Please don't tell my wife.) Additionally, I've never met a person or team member who did their job perfectly.

However, working together with my perfect teams, I built ten high-volume practices, had a ton of fun, and made gobs of money in the process.

In fact, my perfect teams (made up of imperfect people) were such a delight, I loved coming to work. Granted, some days were more work than others, but most days I was hard-pressed to think of anything I'd rather be doing or any place I'd rather be.

It wasn't always that way for me. I struggled like everyone else and wondered some days if it was worth it. Then a career-ending injury and pure necessity put me on a path to discover a process and system that helped me build many perfect teams in those ten high-volume, high-profit offices that delivered great care.

I did it with the following Seven Keys to a Perfect Team.

1. Create templates, then train and cross-train every position.

DCs and all types of CAs perform better when they know the purpose, the tasks of their positions, and what other team members' jobs are. This requires work and consistency, but some management consultant has already put the job descriptions and checklists in a manual you can copy and modify to suit your needs. The trick is to actually do it.

Hot Tip: Role-playing increases certainty and puts your practice on procedure rails. Using patient procedure templates makes the day-to-day work easier and holds the team to the perfect standard.

2. Give feedback.

Start with appreciation for good work and a positive attitude. Express gratitude for consistency, and give correction when needed. If all you give is praise, that's manipulation and reveals a weakness and fear of confrontation.

Hot Tip: Teach the team to give and receive praise from each other at the morning huddle and office meeting.

3. Pay well.

You can't bribe the poor performer to do better work, but you can reward the hard-working, talented people with more money. An extra $2 an hour is only $350 a month. The cost of constantly replacing and retraining is many times that.

Hot Tip: I give a small raise at ninety days if someone masters their job, and I make the second raise at twelve months bigger than they were expecting.

4. Get rid of the troublemakers.

Want to keep good team members? Then fire people who are moody, pouty, grumpy, grouchy, and just no fun to work with. A bad apple will spoil the whole box, and the team will respect and thank you for letting a troublemaker go. The mood will instantly improve, and you'll never miss them. By the way, no one ever fired anyone too early.

Hot Tip: Teams that train regularly find it easy to integrate new hires.

5. Hold regular office meetings where your job is to listen.

The more you talk in your own office meeting, the worse it is. The more the perfect team shares, reports, asks questions, and commends the other team members, the better the meeting.

Hot Tip: At your next office meeting, instruct each person to bring a professional win they made that week, a report on their work, and a compliment for another team member. Everyone shares, and you're only allowed to answer questions at the end.

6. Play by your own rules, and don't play favorites.

Perfect teams thrive when the doctor plays fair, holding themselves to the same rules they expect others to follow.

Hot Tip: Report to your front desk CA like they are your boss. I did that, and it works like magic to build a better team.

7. Give everyone a scorecard.

Teach them to keep their own position statistics. Some staff will think they can't play the game because they don't know what their "score" is. Of course, the score is different for a front desk CA and an associate DC, but everyone needs to know how what they're doing impacts the organization in order to win.

Hot Tip: Collect statistics at least every week, and use them to praise the wins and help the struggling. You'll trade a vague, suspicious atmosphere that hurts a team for a real understanding of your team's strengths and weaknesses. And if your team member isn't interested in helping with their stats, see #4.

When the team is functioning at its best, work is not only enjoyable—it's perfect.

Don't get me wrong; it's still work, but it's also fun. You work your tail off on the ski slopes, on the basketball court, or in the garden, but that's fun, right? This is the same thing. Follow these seven keys, and the perfect team will appear right before your eyes.

Snapshot: The office is full of patients, the phone's ringing, the CAs are busy and smiling, the tables are full, and the flow is steady. The associates are taking great care of their patients and yours exactly the way you've trained them to.

You can hear a new patient being booked by the CA exactly to your scripts and see an associate bringing a patient to the front desk to book their ROF.

You look at the clock and see that you finished your day right on schedule—your front desk CA sees to that. You'll be out on vacation for the next two weeks, and you know your perfect team will handle everything just the way you've trained them to do. And then it hits you.

This is PERFECT.

As you leave that night, your perfect team tells you to relax and have a great holiday while they handle everything—and don't get sunburned.

As you drive away, you know they'll hardly miss you, and there's a twinge. "I'm going to miss this and will love coming back refreshed. *Perfect.*"

40

Cutting Your Staff Management Stress in Half

The biggest stress in an established chiropractic practice is staff management. Working with people is hard, and as I write this, countless client stories pop into my head. I've coached well over one thousand DCs on their staffing issues, after managing ten highly profitable offices of my own. I think I've heard it all.

This associate said this.

The CA won't do that.

You won't believe what the therapy assistant did!

But how is it that some practices have a fraction of the employee problems others have? What do those doctors know that others don't? The following strategies and tips will help you reduce employee problems, uncomfortable confrontations, and the wasted time of rehiring and retraining—only to have to fire again and start again.

First, it's a lot easier to manage when you are leading, so share your vision and goals for the practice with your staff. It's your job as clinic owner to clarify where the practice is going, and it's the staff's job to make the best contribution to your vision. I can tell you CAs long for their doctors to cast a vision for the future. This lets them see how their jobs fit into the big picture. It's clean, honest, and direct.

Second, you can't manage employees if you aren't willing to confront problems. However, you can make confrontation half as hard right off the bat by fixing four common mistakes.

Mistake #1: Failure to outline and discuss *in detail* how each employee needs to treat their job, the practice, patients, and coworkers

Solution: Write your wants, desires, and standards into an employee office policy. Let everyone know what behavior you expect. Have each employee read and sign it. It does not guarantee perfection, but it lays a foundation for successful employee management.

Example: I don't believe facial piercing is appropriate in a chiropractic clinic. I clearly state that in the dress code portion of my office policy. Additionally, I don't want people coming to me to borrow against future paychecks. That's mentioned too.

Mistake #2: Failure to completely outline the employee's job duties

Solution: Write up a *detailed* job description, including the toughest parts of the job and those things that are only done on rare occasions. New hires are typically excited about a new job and are willing to embrace the entire position and all of its responsibilities.

Example: I also include a section at the end of the job description that states that the job description may change without notice based on clinic goals and the needs of the practice. I explain that concept carefully and have the employee sign it.

Mistake #3: Failure to see that "being nice" is poor management.

Some doctors tell me they're just too nice to be effective managers, but the truth isn't that they're too nice. "Too nice" is code for fear of confrontation. When you fail to confront or feel compelled to give in to an employee who needs correction, it isn't being *nice*—it's bad management.

Never think that ignoring bad behavior will eliminate it. It sanctions it instead.

Here's how poor management compounds your stress: If you let a rule slide three times (because you're "too nice") you have created new policy and given the signal that the boss is powerless. You end up asking, "I'm so nice; why do they take advantage of me?" The answer is *because* you're too nice.

A client told me that he cured himself of being too nice with a simple mental adjustment. He substitutes the word *weak* for *nice*. He hates being weak, and just thinking about his behavior differently gave him the right attitude to make the right choice.

Solution: If an employee problem is based on a knowledge or a procedure problem, then retrain. If it's an attitude problem, take them back to the signed office policy and/or job description.

Example: "We clearly outlined this in the office policy and in your job description. The person who has your position must show up on time (or whatever the infraction). If that person is you, you need to start showing up on time now. If you can't be here on time, you need to tell me now." The ball is in their court. If they can't be on time, find someone who will. It may be hard, but it's that simple.

Mistake #4: Failure to provide ongoing training for every position in the office.

Any staff member can get off track or forget who the boss is if you don't consistently train—even after they know the position.

Solution: Schedule and prioritize weekly office meetings where you role-play and run drills.

Example: I built a chain of very profitable chiropractic offices that run like little Swiss watches because I am committed to training and checking up on performance. Remember, you don't get what you expect—you get what you train for and continue to inspect.

Live by these rules, and you'll have a fraction of your current employee stress and enjoy your practice much more than you do now.

41

Secrets for Developing the Best Front Desk CA Ever

I stood at the front desk counting end-of-day numbers: eight new patients and 136 regular visits for three chiropractors, and half that for physical and massage therapies. All in all, it had been a good (busy) day, and every visit had been handled expertly by my front desk CA (FDCA).

I looked up as Claudine, my FDCA for the past eighteen months, handed me all the stats as she dashed for the door. "Gotta go. Mostly good. I'll give feedback at the huddle. See you then, good night," she said with a sincere smile. It was 6:12 p.m. —just minutes after the last patient left—and Claudine was rushing to get Philip from day care.

I looked at her workstation: almost everything perfectly neat except for Claudine's work pile that she would coordinate with the biller in the morning.

Everyone at the practice liked Claudine, and I was crazy about her. She ran my office at 600-720 visits a week, just like a Swiss watch—mainly because I planned it that way.

Here are my secrets for empowering a FDCA to be your best team member.

First, let's take a look at a front desk CA's job duties: scheduling, greeting, routing, and taking payments. Your FDCA controls the flow of the entire clinic. From their vantage point, they can see the schedule, the reception area, and frequently the patient care areas.

So tell me, who's the best person to give the orders concerning who goes where and when? Is it the DC, who may be behind closed doors and struggling to keep track of time? No, it's your FDCA. They're in the perfect position to quarterback the team, cut your stress in half, and take real ownership of their position.

Hot Tip: Train a strong front desk CA to run your office exactly how you want it run, then give them the whip. Then learn phrases like "Yes, ma'am/sir!" and "Where do you need me next?"

Here's my thinking: I work for the goals of my chiropractic clinic. I know that as the owner, I get to set those goals, but as a treating doctor, I also work for them.

Once I have shared my goals and vision for the practice with my front desk CA and told them exactly how each team member needs to function in order to reach those goals, then I should give them the responsibility and authority to direct the process. My job is to bust my tail to be the best team member under the FDCA's direction.

I work for my front desk CA, and Claudine was a demanding boss. One of my associates—a man who hated being told what to do by anyone, but especially a woman—once complained, "Dr. Lloyd, you let her boss you around!"

Just to be clear, Claudine was direct in her communication but never rude or disrespectful to anyone, especially me, and the results were amazing.

"I don't mind being 'bossed around' by someone who bosses as well as she does," I told the associate. "And by the way, her boss"—and here I pointed to myself— "trained her and is thrilled with how she runs this place."

Do you want your FDCA engaged and excited about the job? Do you want them to take ownership of their position? Do you want your FDCA to take care of your practice like it was their own?

Then the secret is to outline the game, explain the rules, give them authority and responsibility to run the practice, and play your position like it's the Super Bowl and they're the coach. The synergy is exciting, and the work is a fraction of what it might be now.

Here are my five secrets for empowering your FDCA to be your best team member in the best way ever.

1. Share your practice vision and patient care goals with a strong FDCA.

Not all people can do this position well, so pick a good one with a strong work ethic, who cares about the job, and then train them well and train them often.

Hot Tip: This process of recruiting their heart to your vision requires an ongoing dialogue about what you're trying to build as part of their training. Ask for and listen to their feedback.

2. Agree to play by the rules you set up, and ask them to hold you to it.

This won't work if your ego is too fragile to take strong direction. For best results, lead by example. Insist your associates and other team members comply, and then seek feedback from your FDCA. "How'd we do today, Claudine?"

Hot Tip: Your willingness to play by your own rules is very motivating for your FDCA. They can also become your cheerleader (not babysitter) and help you stay focused throughout the day.

3. Set up the authority and responsibility of the FDCA for the entire team.

Gather everyone in an office meeting where the FDCA explains your shared practice vision, shared goals, and each task in their job description.

After that, invite each staff person to ask the FDCA this scripted question: "What do you need from me for you to run the team at peak performance? Tell me *everything* you need from me, and I promise I'll do my best."

As everyone asks the question, take notes on what the FDCA says and repeat it back to them for clarity. And yes, you should take your turn with the script too. Remember, follow your own rules and lead by example.

Hot Tip: Instruct the FDCA to publicly acknowledge exceptional service from teammates at the next day's morning huddle.

4. Call a morning huddle fifteen minutes before patients arrive.

The whole crew should gather around the day's schedule as you announce, "Claudine is going to tell us what she needs from us today."

The FDCA might run a huddle like this:

"First, everyone functioned extremely well yesterday. A special thanks to Katie for her help during power hours, and Dr. Kane's overflow coverage was right on time. We rocked it!

"Now, today's fairly busy, but we have a normal morning until 10:00 a.m., when I've booked three new patients followed by four ROFs, and then a busy late morning. I'll need Dr. Lloyd finished with all adjustments and ready to take the Smiths back for health histories at 10:00 a.m. sharp. Dr. Sanders, you'll start your new patient at the same time in Exam Room 2."

Hot Tip: It takes time for an FDCA to grow into the job the way you want it done. Be patient and strengthen their skills by telling them what to look for and complimenting good insight and decisions. When the day has run smoothly, thank them.

5. Keep the FDCA job streamlined.

Resist the temptation to pile on tasks that require your FDCA to leave the front desk. If they're dashing back to take someone off therapy every ten minutes, a simple job can become chaotic. And when the FDCA is pressured, they don't produce or handle flow well. Keep them at the front desk with as few back-office distractions as possible. Fill the time between patients with flow-related tasks to increase volume, such as inactive recalls to fill the gaps in the schedule.

Hot Tip: When the DC needs help, use an associate who can not only be the doctor's clinical assistant but also adjust overflow, produce their own new patients, and generate income for the clinic.

To have a successful practice that purrs like a kitten, even at high volume, we need more than tasks checked off on a checklist. We need motivated, engaged, and empowered CAs and associates in every position of the clinic.

Use my five-point plan to empower other positions with responsibility and authority as well. Before you know it, you'll have an entire team of superstar performers trained and eager to create your vision and reach your practice goals.

42

Hiring and Firing Dos and Don'ts

Dr. Nick loved his chiropractic practice, but this morning he dreaded his drive to work.

For months, he'd needed to fire his front desk CA but hadn't.

This wasn't the first time Nick had trouble letting someone go. In fact, he had a pattern. He hired in a hurry and scrimped on training. When he was lucky, the new employee would catch on and hang in there. More often, the situation soured, and he found himself paying a person who needed to go.

It gets worse. Nick also had trouble giving employees encouragement or correction. Eventually, their mistakes made him angry, and he would end up hating their work but unable to fire them. He'd tell himself the following:

"It's my fault. I haven't trained her like I should've."

"Patients are crazy about him!"

"She used to do great work."

"Who'd do the job if I fired him?"

"Can't fire her today; we're too busy."

"I'll give him one more chance."

Deep down, he knew these were just excuses, but he didn't have the skills to face the problem today.

Nick's not alone. This story is repeated every day in chiropractic practices around the world.

Why is firing a person so hard? You hire people when there's work to do and say good-bye when they can't or won't do the work. It sounds simple, doesn't it? It isn't.

In fact, hiring, managing, and firing people is the biggest stressor in an established practice. If you're a practice owner, you'll always be hiring or firing someone.

My advice is get used to it and get good at it.

My Epiphany

Years ago, I owned five busy practices, a marketing company, and Five Star, my management and consulting company. I was literally hiring and firing on a weekly basis.

I remember the point when I suddenly understood that the comings and goings of employees were normal. Letting someone go wasn't personal. We just weren't a good fit.

Firing wasn't fun, but if I fired well, everyone felt better— maybe not immediately, but soon. This realization allowed me to hire and fire with a clearer head and very little negative emotion.

I'm guessing you're better at staff development than our fictitious Dr. Nick, but sooner or later, you'll need to let someone go. Here are the guidelines I still use today to make the process of hiring and firing easier on everyone.

Hiring

You'd like to have the right person do great work for a long time, so hire well.

1. Define the work you want done in a clear job description with a complete checklist of each task for the position. This will make it easier to find your next superstar.

2. When I hire CAs, I begin with a group informational meeting, where I save time by explaining the job and team standards to between four and twelve prospects at a time. I administer written tests and follow with private interviews to select our finalists.

3. I invite the top one or two applicants back for a working interview, where they observe and participate in a paid job audition. Do they engage? After two hours, are they still excited to step into the position? How will they work with us and our patients?

4. I check all references, Google each applicant's name, check their social media profiles, and run a formal background check.

5. As a final selector, I use Nordstrom's axiom: "Hire the smile, train the skill."

   I look more for potential than experience and seek to hire the rising star who I can train in my systems and procedures.

I never hire someone who would have an uncomfortably long commute, or the person who used to earn more than I'm offering, or someone who's had three or more jobs in the last two years.

Hot Tip: You can increase your chances of a good hire by putting your new employee into a comprehensive training program.

Firing

When should you fire an employee? I've never met an employer who felt they fired a problem employee too early, and most people will say they fired too late. If you think it might be time, it usually is.

Example #1: The nice, friendly person who can't do the work.
You've given them their twelfth chance. Not all people can do this
kind of work, and if the job is beyond a person's capability, let
them go. The right person can do the work easily.

**Example #2: The person who won't do the work—the one
with the attitude.** It's definitely time to bid this employee farewell.
Life's too short to work with people looking for an argument.
You'll be amazed what patients will tell you about this person
after they're gone.

**Example #3: The employee you catch telling lies, cheating,
or stealing.** They need to be let go ASAP. You may even need to
contact the police, but check with your attorney first.

If you start to notice examples #1 and #2, try at first to make
the relationship work with extra training, verbal warnings, and
written warnings. However, when you know it's not going to work,
let them go. Keeping bad employees, even if they're nice people,
can demotivate your team and make the practice miserable for
everyone.

When it's time to fire, use these guidelines:

1. Fire when the time is right for you—whether that's at the end
   of the month, week, or typically the end of the person's shift.
2. Set the stage for the termination meeting. "Gina, at the end
   of your shift meet me in my office, please."
3. Have another staff person act as a witness at the termination
   to protect your position.
4. Never make a firing personal. If you're angry, you waited too
   long. Never give a fired employee a reason to seek revenge.
5. Keep it short and sweet. "Gina, I need a different result in our
   marketing program, and I've decided to rehire your position.
   I'm letting you go effective immediately. Would you like me
   to explain why?" (They usually know why.) "I'm sure you'll

do well elsewhere, and I wish you the best. Brittany will take your key and help you with your things."

Hot Tip: Before they're out of the parking lot, change all their passwords and never—and I mean never—hire them back. Make no exceptions.

Don't bad-mouth a fired employee to remaining staff. It's beneath you.

You may need to scramble to fill a position, but that's a smaller problem than letting a bad employee linger, and I promise your drive to the office will be pleasant again—except for the traffic.

43

Tenure Versus Merit

I've heard more than my share of chiropractors complain about their staff. In fact, the staffing issue is the biggest stress for established practices with over one hundred visits a week. (If you're under one hundred visits a week, your biggest stress is how to get *over* one hundred visits a week.)

The truth is, working with people can be difficult, but it will be a lot less difficult if you understand the best way to handle their first few days, and how to make your expectations crystal clear from the start.

I owe this discussion to my friend and business associate Dr. George Birnbach. Ever since I heard him explain it, I've had the following conversation with every staff member, and it's saved me countless headaches.

As a short aside, I know that most chiropractic offices struggle greatly with employee launching and follow-up training. I often hear, "I don't know how to do a launch or train, Noel!"—and this comment is from the honest doctors. The clueless ones just think the problem is in the pool of applicants.

Few DCs have an established weekly training time or even anything in the office with "new employee essentials" (or a similar phrase) written on it.

Most employee launches are just two words: "Good luck!" Follow-up training is three words: "Hang in there!" Is it a wonder that chiropractic practices have the turnover they do?

Contrast that with the thousands of successful businesses that identify their new employee orientation and follow-up training procedures as the top reason for the company's success, and you start to see staff launch and follow-up training in perspective.

The following is a key piece of my launch and integration script for my practice and management company. You can use this for new or established employees right out of the box.

Here's the setting: It's an orientation meeting between the owner (me) and a new employee. We're sitting in my office, and I'm explaining my part of how to be a successful employee at Sound Chiropractic Centers.

Owner: "Can you tell me what tenure means?"

Employee: "Isn't that what professors get?"

Owner: "You're right, but what does it mean?"

Employee: "Not sure, but it protects the employee's job, right?"

Owner: "Exactly. What tenure means is that your employer can't change your position or the conditions of employment without extraordinary circumstances.

"Now, can you tell me what a merit-based job is?"

Employee: "I'm guessing here, but it probably means the employee has to earn his or her position, right?"

Owner: "You're exactly right. The employee is evaluated based on the merit of their work in the position. Now, tell me—is my job a tenured position or a merit position?"

Employee: "You own the company, so I guess you're tenured, right?"

Owner: "Wrong. I'm merit. Every private business owner is paid in the strictest sense in a merit system. Did you know that the overwhelming percentage of small businesses go broke? The mortality, or death rate, is 80 percent in the first five years, and almost as high in the next five years. In short, we're here because I've worked my tail off.

"Now, tell me—is *your* job tenure or merit?"

Employee: "I bet it's merit, isn't it?"

Owner: "Exactly. Merit, and like my job, it always will be. You can do brilliant work for ten years, but if you decide that you want to start coasting on your reputation, you and I'll be done—just like that.

"Does that sound harsh?"

Employee: "Not really. I think I get it."

Owner: "That doesn't mean that you can't earn loyalty. That's built on reputation. If you earn a good reputation as a hard worker we can count on for reliable, consistent work, and who's willing to go the extra mile, then I'll support you to the hilt.

"Now, let's go over the goals of the clinic and your position again, and I'll explain how your job fits into the big picture here. I'll outline the stats I'll have you keep, explain your training schedule, and make some assignments. Does that make sense? Super."

What I've just done in a fair and kind way is let my new hire know that I work hard and expect that they will too. I also let them know that I'll measure their merit with the organization objectively (through statistics) and that I'll train them to do good work so they can earn merit and a good reputation. I've also explained that time spent with the company doesn't mean security, but merit and a good reputation will mean they'll always have my strong support.

Hot Tip: Read this chapter with your staff and ask for a reaction. It'll help you lower your stress, put you back in the driver's seat, and make practice more fun again.

44

Make the Most of Office Meetings

I used to hate office meetings, and now I love them. What changed?

I now believe the office meeting was the single most important tool I had for running my ten offices smoothly and at a high profit.

The purpose of the office meeting is communication. Though smaller offices (two or three people) communicate throughout the week as a function of working together, they still need an office meeting. Structured meeting communication is different.

A good chiropractic office meeting is designed around the activities that make an office function the way it should—high energy, low stress, and a lot of fun. These activities are seldom done outside a structured meeting, and they include:

- Information
- Inspiration
- Execution
- Education
- Demonstration

Information

Everyone needs to know where the business is and where it's headed. A simple restating of the stats and goals of the clinic or office is the first step. Office meetings are the place to discuss the details—the *who*, *what*, *why*, *how*, and *when* of each addition or change in the office. This lets the staff see what you want and how you think. The information phase is both foundational *and* motivational. Higher motivation for your staff is a side effect of the informing process.

An old Estée Lauder ad stated, "Knowing is everything." Industrial psychologists tell us that "knowing" or "being on the inside" when it comes to information about their work is more important to your staff than pay issues.

The other side of that card is that it's not motivating to be the last to know. Imagine trying to feel like you're a valued team member making a contribution, only to end up hearing everything about your office and position secondhand.

Basic information can be both important and interesting. How did we do? What are our practice goals, and are we achieving them? What new programs are we implementing and why? How can I help? How are you feeling? How are the patients doing?

Inspiration

Your office meeting should inspire. Properly motivated people are more important to your office than properly trained people. In fact, motivation is the single most important issue for a doctor and staff. Most of us have employed brilliant people who were an absolute menace and less stellar individuals we remember fondly because they had such a great attitude. Inspiration and motivation are inseparable and vital to your success.

Execution

This is where you discuss all projects past, present, and future. We evaluate the past, activate the present, and plan the future. At the end of this chapter, I have included a sample agenda from one of my own office meetings so that you see what I mean.

Education

The largest restaurant chain in the world has made billions of hamburgers—and dollars—with an unskilled labor force of varying quality. Can we really credit the food for such tremendous success? No, McDonald's maintains the highest standards of reproducible quality in their industry through a commitment to staff education and training that borders on obsessive.

The more we know about something, the better we can deal with it. That hasn't escaped the best companies around the world—industry leaders—who all seem to be equally obsessed with education.

Demonstration

There's just one way you can truly know for sure that you or anyone else can do a particular task or activity, and that's to witness it demonstrated firsthand. Every time I hear a DC or CA say, "Yeah, we do that," or "I already know how to do that," without offering details, I'm willing to bet even money they don't do it.

Never believe it until you see it role-played, by memory, and word perfect.

Cynical or smart? Smart. My opinion has been forged in the hot fire of working with support staff and associate doctors over decades. There's no value judgment here; it's just the way you and I and every other person need to be managed.

Preparing for Your Meeting

- Have a purpose.
- Have a time.
- Have a place.
- Have a leader.
- Have a secretary.
- Have an agenda.
- Have some rules:
  - Do the work required for the meeting before the meeting.
  - Start and end on time.
  - Stick to the agenda.
  - Minimize interruptions.
  - Require that everyone participate.
  - Bring a problem, bring a solution. If you need help with a problem that must be shared at the meeting, you must also propose a solution to your own problems.
  - Don't do committee work in a meeting.
- Don't expect perfection at first.

Sample Five Star Office Meeting Agenda (one hour)

I.   Statistics Review for the Practice
  A. Weekly Statistics
  B. Monthly Statistics
  C. Year-to-Date Statistics
II. New Practice Records and Goal Setting
III. Wins (everyone MUST bring a win)
IV. Past: Completed Event/Project Evaluation
  A. What happened?
  B. Did we reach our objectives?
  C. What went right?

      D. What went wrong?

      E. What would we do differently?

      F. Who do we need to thank/acknowledge?

  V. Present: Current Event/Project Progress Reviews

      A. Action taken?

      B. Action needed?

      C. Action blocked?

  VI. Future: New Projects

      A. What?

      B. Why?

      C. Who?

      D. How?

      E. When?

  VII. Chiropractic Education (staff picks topics)

VIII. Patient Testimonies/Progress

  IX. Office Procedure

      A. Role-play last assigned procedure(s)

      B. Review new procedure(s)

      C. Assign reading and memory work in notes

      D. Deadline for new procedure(s)

  X. Closing

      A. Review decisions and assignments

      B. Questions

45

Thirty Minutes That Will Revolutionize Your Office

A DC client took one of their CAs to a seminar, only to have her miss the meetings because she was hungover and ill in her hotel room after partying late the night before. Her behavior crashed the entire weekend for his team, and she lost her job as a result.

You've probably heard this kind of story, or perhaps you experienced something like this yourself. It's a big disappointment, and an even bigger waste.

But that's nothing compared to the thousands of doctors who squander an *entire year* of seminars full of excellent information, motivation, team building, and resultant practice growth just by not preparing themselves or their staff for training.

How big of a waste is this really? Think of all your hard-earned money in the back of an open pickup truck speeding down the highway. Some of that cash is bound to stick to something, but most of it is lost. Scary enough for you?

I'm going to give you my secrets and a simple strategy for a thirty-minute meeting that will maximize the effect of any seminar you attend with your staff. In fact, the whole point here is to help you extract every dollar of information, motivation, and momentum that you pay for... and a lot you don't.

How good are these secrets? I developed two associates to over five hundred visits a week, another group of four to more than 390 a week, and four of my ten offices went over three hundred visits a week with just one DC, one full-time CA, and one part-time CA each.

So let's go.

First, if it happens in *your* practice, *you're* responsible. If you're not, who is? Our friend with the wild CA needed to let her know what acceptable behavior looks like. But I'm talking about much more than acceptable behavior. I'm talking about exceptional performance.

Second, if you're responsible for what happens in your practice, you're also responsible for what your staff gets out of seminars. Therefore, you need to train and prepare your staff to not only behave well but to gain all they can from special training.

For example, if you hunt, fish, ski, or go boating, the success of your outing hinges on preparation. If you don't plan, you may not have the right clothes, the right equipment, or enough gas, and you could be in big trouble.

I learned this lesson one weekend when I got in my neighbor's boat to travel from a remote island to the mainland during high winds. He told me everything would be fine. However, just as we were taking every other wave over the bow, he ran out of gas. By God's grace, we were rescued. Now I always take responsibility to check all the gas tanks on every boat trip.

How does this apply to what I'm discussing here? I bring all my DCs and CAs to seminars and have for decades. Done right, it's a great investment. Yet I quickly learned that "done right" meant I needed to prepare my staff for the best results.

In prepping for a seminar, I ask DCs and CAs alike for written answers and discussion of the following questions:

- What is your vision for your position (ask again, even if it's for the umpteenth time), and how does it serve the chiropractic vision?
- What does your position look, sound, and feel like when things are working as well as they can? During our power hours?
- What are your three biggest position wins so far this year?
- What are your three biggest position challenges right now?
- What are three things you want for your position from the upcoming seminar?
- What is your strategy for getting the most from the upcoming event?
- What are your action steps for reaching your goals?

I encourage each individual to participate in the seminar by asking questions of the speakers—especially asking the top experts in attendance how they handle key issues—and introducing themselves to the leader types and other sharp DCs and CAs in attendance.

I tell my staff members they will need to take and organize notes and quotes for our debriefing meeting that will follow when we get back to the office, as each person will be teaching me what they learned. By doing this, I'm protecting my investment, empowering my staff, and enlisting them to help me reach clinic goals.

The debriefing meeting is an excellent management tool. Just by scheduling the meeting before we leave for the seminar, staff members know they'll have to contribute, and that usually means they pay better attention during the training. I applaud good contributions and initiative, as well as listen for what's missing. Typically, I'll incorporate at least part of everyone's ideas in our plans going forward, which has produced an invested and motivated staff.

As for seminar conduct, I have a little speech:

"We're going to the seminar to learn, have fun, and share. We want to better ourselves and extract ideas that will make it easier to serve chiropractic, help people, have more fun, and be more successful. You can't do that hungover or without sleep. You represent this practice so be reasonable and get enough sleep to do your best work.

"It's up to you to get your answers and solutions; so listen, take notes, ask questions, and mingle with the best and brightest during the breaks.

"Now, each of you tell me what you're going to bring back to the office and share at the debriefing meeting....

"Great, let's go."

46

Exactly This, Exactly This Way

You've worked hard, acquired skills, persevered, built a practice, got busy, and then discovered that not only do you have a successful practice, but a successful practice has you.

This is never more apparent than when you need to take a sick day or want to take a vacation. Good-bye, three to ten thousand dollars.

So you hire an associate with the hope of working side-by-side with someone who "gets it." But they don't get it. In fact, they don't get many things right at all.

Their lack of "get it" shows up as few or no new patients and terrible patient retention You worry about having them adjust even one of your patients, let alone cover a sick day or—God forbid—a vacation.

Ah, but there's more, and it's worse. Now you're making less money—a lot less money. "How in the world did I end up here?" you ask.

This exact scenario was described to me by a sharp, successful DC during what Five Star calls a Test Drive.

I asked why he was so upset. "Did you ever tell your associate expressly and exactly what you wanted and when?"

"I shouldn't have to. He should have known!"

"How's that working for you?" I asked. He paused, and then all his defensiveness left as he laughed the words, "It ain't."

Then he asked me what I'd do.

Here's the key piece I want you to take away from this story: I told him he had no right to expect anything that wasn't on a checklist, clearly explained, agreed upon, and trained for. I explained a phrase my associates all know well:

"Do EXACTLY this, EXACTLY this way."

Think of how clueless you were when you got out of school. Now make a list of all the great things you've learned over the years, including the scripts, care protocols, answers to patient questions—everything.

Now write it all down on a checklist. Script it out where needed, and then explain to your associate *why you do it that way* and train them to do it *exactly that way.*

The doctor I was talking to had an interesting response to my suggestion. "That doesn't seem too respectful of a colleague, does it?"

I told him that an associate doesn't hire on for respect. They come because they want training. You want immediate results.

You'll both get what you want if you create a template for everything you want them to get and then train to that template.

47

How to Lose Tons of Money

Dr. Mike wanted to increase his income by increasing patient services, so he added massage therapy, a popular weight-loss program, and a chiropractic associate. With insurance reimbursements down, he thought offering more services would be a great way to boost collections. Plus, Mike liked the fact he wouldn't have to personally provide the new services.

Mike had another idea. He'd open the office on Friday afternoon and Saturday morning.

The clinic will finally make money without me actually being there, he thought.

The net result? Mike doubled his stress and took home $51,000 *less* than the year before.

Wait a minute! Mike added services that he billed for, increased the service time, and LOST take-home dollars? Yep, Mike lost a big chunk of his profit and ended up working a lot harder—definitely not what the doctor ordered.

Mike's not alone. Every month I speak to smart, successful docs who've added services and personnel, only to lose money.

The good news is it doesn't have to be that way. Add services the right way, and your patients will love it, your staff will do the hands-on work, and you'll profit handsomely.

So where did Mike go wrong? I've been guiding people through this process for more than twenty-five years, and when it crashes, it's usually because of the same set of mistakes. Let's take a look at each misstep and give Dr. Mike some solutions.

Mistake #1: Not treating each additional service as a separate business that needs to produce a profit

Here's how even smart docs like Mike get fooled. He was already making good money and thought that adding extra services would be easy. The programs would just catch on.

The term "catch on" is code for "I've got no plan." And no plan is a plan to fail.

Solution: Add just one carefully launched service at a time, and even then, do it only after drawing up what I call a street-smart business plan. This real-life strategy sheet needs to clearly outline how you're going to build your business into profit ASAP. Remember to calculate all of the costs—especially labor.

Another critical page is the marketing plan. You need solid answers to the two most important questions in any practice: *How do we get new patients or clients and who's going to get them?*

Mistake #2: Not having one primary person to implement the business plan for each service

The last thing Mike needed was a bunch of extra projects on top of his current jobs as staff trainer, staff manager, marketing manager, office bookkeeper, and full-time chiropractor. There was no way he could keep on top of new services too.

In retrospect, Mike's de facto management strategy was the all-too-common "throw it against the wall and see if it sticks." Things were not sticking.

Solution: Each area of service in your chiropractic practice needs one person to lead the project. The project lead needs to understand Mike's vision and be able to implement his plan for how the service will be delivered. They also must know they're accountable for how the plan is working.

For Mike, his project leads would be his massage therapist, the weight-loss specialist, and his associate who covered the weekend hours.

Mistake #3: Not having accurate and up-to-the-minute stats

Without concrete data or statistics to tell him how each new service was producing, Mike was flying blind. He thought things looked busier, but the only real information he saw was weeks after the program launches, when he pulled his profit and loss statement only to see he'd taken home less money for yet another month.

Solution: Every project lead should report in three very important ways.

First report: The project leads provide a live sixty-second check-in and check-out *every day.* Each project lead should find Mike first thing in the morning and fill him in on what part of the business plan and marketing they're working on that day. At the end of the day, the project lead checks out by reporting what got accomplished. Together, the in and out takes two minutes per person.

Second report: The project leads either hand, email, or text their daily stats to Mike every day.

Third report: The project leads bring their weekly stats to the office meeting, where they report to the whole team how their services are progressing.

With these three reports, Mike would have known in real time what was being done and how it affected his bank account. He could have made corrections or changes to his plan based on solid information.

Let me share a real-life example. Dr. Phil (no, not that one) has multiple services, or *businesses* as we call them, both inside and outside his office. Here's what Phil gets every day from each of his businesses:

His in-office personnel each catch him for a short (sixty-second) check-in as the day begins. That includes his two associates, one massage therapist, and the CA who runs the weight-loss program. A project lead from an outside business has already called him on his mobile with her check-in.

As Dr. Phil says, "It's great! In the first ten to fifteen minutes of my day I know what every project lead is thinking and what they believe needs to be done."

At the end of the day, project leads are responsible for tracking Dr. Phil down for a check-out that takes less than a minute each. He squares what they tell him with what they promised that morning, and all is good. Or, if not, he asks questions as he looks over his stats on their Post-it notes.

Net result? Phil's in the loop in the best possible way, the businesses are running well, and he's making money.

Next, at the religiously consistent weekly office meeting, Dr. Phil listens to each project lead report their stats, wins, and near-term goals to the team. He truly is in control of every phase of the practice and each income stream.

Oh, I almost forgot. Do you remember Mike's decision to extend his hours? Typically, that's a huge mistake. His clinic didn't see more patients. They just spread their existing visits over more hours, which had to be covered by support staff, which drove up his labor costs. He should have waited until the associate's practice required more room or clinic hours.

Now for a quick review of how to add new services and NOT lose money:

1. Launch one service at a time, using a street-smart business plan to be in profit ASAP.
2. Appoint one person as project lead of each service.
3. Require daily check-in, check-out, and stat reports. It's their responsibility to find you. Don't chase them.
4. Project leads share weekly stats at the office meeting.
5. Keep new services limited to normal hours to keep your eye on them and save labor costs.

48

The Successful Chiropractor's Dirty Little Secret

You love chiropractic, love your patients, and love your busy, successful practice. You're the envy of colleagues, friends, and neighbors.

But I know your dirty little secret. As great as your practice is, you're chained to it. And, if you try to sneak away—even for a short time—it can cost you tens of thousands of dollars. You're a prisoner.

Here's what I mean: You take your family of four to Europe, the Caribbean, or Hawaii for one short week. Depending on how you fly, where you stay, and what you do when you get there (don't forget the shopping), it can cost $12,000 to $15,000, right?

Wrong, and you know where this is going, don't you?

The price of the trip is only half the cost. You lose *another* $12,000 to $15,000 in practice revenue for being out of the office.

And then, instead of a packed schedule when you return, the practice seems to have "hurt feelings," and it takes a little time and TLC to get back to its old, sweet, affectionate self. The total damages could exceed $30,000.

A philosophical approach would be that it all evens out, but it's expensive. And isn't this why you've become the master of the three- or four-day weekend vacation? I've met many DCs who haven't had a full week off in a decade or more. A few have good vacation relief help, but most lose money and patients when they're out of the office.

How many of you are thinking about a full two weeks off, or a solid month of freedom? Didn't think so.

In short, you're a slave to your success. Don't get me wrong. If this is your stress, you have it good. Many DCs struggle in their practice their entire lives and would give their eyeteeth for your day-to-day life and income. But you're still a prisoner. The handcuffs are gold, but they're still handcuffs.

Good news! It doesn't have to be that way. You can have more freedom, a better income, and a practice that greets you with a kiss at the door when you return after an enjoyable vacation.

Here's an example: Dr. John loves his practice. He's also a big NASCAR fan and takes his family to key races in their motorhome. On a race week, he'll leave town Wednesday night and not return to the office until Tuesday morning. John also takes several full weeks off each year. Just ask him about Hawaii.

And by the way, John is doing yet another best-ever year in practice.

More freedom AND a better income? How does he do it?

John learned to develop associate doctors the right way.

I can hear it already. "I've had associates before and... (insert negative complaint here)."

I know, I know. Associates are unmotivated and unskilled, feel that the world owes them, and don't appreciate anything you do for them, etc.

The fact is, both sides of the owner-associate equation are often anywhere from cautious to cynical about the arrangement. That shouldn't be a surprise, since most associateships end badly. And, like a bad marriage, each side blames the other.

With so much opportunity and the need so great on both sides, though, why aren't more successful chiropractors developing successful associates in win-win relationships? Who's to blame?

In my twenty-five years of coaching on this subject, I'd say it's usually the owner's fault, but if that's you, that's good news. You can't fix what isn't your fault.

In the next few paragraphs, I'll give you the strategies and systems that have taken me years to piece together and have allowed me to successfully develop dozens of associates and sell ten clinics to associates in real win-win relationships.

First, know that all associates want to succeed and some have the talent and work ethic necessary to do just that—so pick a good one. The best question I ask in my interviews is, "What do you want to be doing in five years?" If their goals don't match yours, walk away.

Second, frame the game correctly for maximum motivation for both of you. I tell associate applicants, "This isn't just a job—it's a career opportunity. Even though I'm the boss, you aren't just working for me—you're working for your future. Whatever your dream practice looks like is what you're working for."

Third, take the time to teach your associate what they really want and are motivated to learn—how to be as successful as you are. Teach the step-by-step nuts and bolts of your success. This is usually where things start to break down—practice owners rarely train their associates enough and, by default, don't lead.

I set aside two hours every Monday to train my associates on every phase of my chiropractic practice's success, starting with marketing, patient management, and patient care.

If you're not sure what to teach your associate, here are two simple strategies:

1. Drag out your favorite consultant's notes, update them with the changes you've added, and teach that.

2. Go high tech, and ask a CA to video you from a patient's point of view as you go through your Day One, Day Two, returning visit, reevaluations, and re-reports. You'll capture exactly what you want your associate to replicate, including scripting, inflection, and even facial expression.

Use a simple video-editing program like iMovie, and you could end up with a series of short videos of key patient interactions—the doctor's greeting, initial history, exam and X-rays, report of findings, etc.—all broken up into short, bite-sized clips.

Don't overthink it—just shoot it. Don't like it? Shoot it again.

You can also narrate a series of short how-to videos about taking and analyzing X-rays, how you arrive at a diagnosis, how to write up a care plan, and how to interface with key CA positions. And wouldn't it be helpful to have a number of short videos on proper use of your computerized chart note system? Store the videos in a learning library on your server, on a training computer, or in a shared file in the cloud. Explain that the associate's goal should be to replicate what they see on the video.

Don't be afraid of hearing your associate parrot your scripts and patient interactions—pray for it.

Marketing is another important topic to share with associates, starting on their first day. If they can produce their own new patients, everything works better. If you and your associate work hard, they'll start to get busy with new patients they produce.

Even if you do everything here, be careful about taking too much time off too soon. When you know your associate can handle it, have them take care of your practice on a Friday. Sometime later, have them cover a Thursday and a Friday, while you slip away for a long weekend. Gradually stretch it out as you trust the results. Eventually, you'll get to this place:

I woke to a knock on my door at 7:05 a.m. Room service had sent my hot black coffee as my wake-up. On the tray was an envelope. I sipped my coffee as I walked to the balcony. The tropical sky, palm trees, and beach looked inviting.

I pulled up a chair on my lanai and opened the envelope. The fax simply read "2,008!!!"

My interoffice manager was letting me know that the practice had seen over 2,000 visits in one week, while I was over six thousand miles away in Palau's Rock Islands on a two-week scuba diving trip.

49

Turning the $188,000 Mistake into Gold

Have all the credit card statements come in yet? Have you run the math? What I'm talking about is your last family vacation.

Perhaps you normally produce and/or collect $10,000 a week from your 160+ patient visits. But not when you take the family on a weeklong vacation to wherever. Bye-bye, $10,000.

You also spent $10,000 on flights, hotels, meals, entertainment, gifts, etc. So now you're out $20,000.

"But I have a great vacation-relief doc!" Super. Now check the practice drop in visits against what you paid the locum, and it's probably the same $20,000 loss.

Actually, it's worse than that. The average practice that's seeing over 160 patient visits a week—because of lost marketing opportunities and a tightening appointment schedule—will also lose another $12,000 *minimum* in missed new patients and patient services.

Let's total the damages. Just two weeks of vacation a year (at $20,000 each) *plus* the $12,000 you're losing each month in missed business, and there's $188,000 down the toilet.

You get to choose. Keep hemorrhaging the $188,000 and be held captive by your success or help more people, have more fun (more freedom), *and* make more money.

What's the solution? No vacations? Pushing yourself to fifty hours a week before and after a big trip?

No. You'll love my idea; I promise. I'm going to outline a course of action that's truly the success strategy that took me from a disabled chiropractor, wondering if I'd be out of practice in a few months, to a managing doctor overseeing two thousand visits a week.

I'm going to break this up into beliefs and actions.

First, believe these things.

1. At over 160 visits a week, you need an associate, even if you think you can see twice that number of patients easily.
2. You can find an associate who will be thrilled to learn from you.
3. You can train your associate to market for new patients.
4. Your associate can collect more than they cost you in fewer than sixty days.
5. Properly trained, your associate, staff, and patients can set records in your absence.

"If the associate succeeds too well, they'll leave me." Maybe, but I have dozens of clients with top-producing associates who stay for more than a decade because they're succeeding and because they know their clinic director has their best interest at heart. They believe they're doing better as an associate than they would on their own.

Second, take action.

In preparation for an associate who'll break clinic records in your absence, do the following:

1. Create templates for your Day One, Day Two, returning visit, reexam/re-X-ray, and New Patient Orientation class procedures including teachable checklists. Then polish your execution of your own checklists. This will be your associate training program and will make practice more fun.

2. Plan out seven to ten hours of external marketing that your associate will do each week to build a practice next to yours. *This is a key step.* If your associate just feeds off your new patients, it's a recipe for disaster.

3. When hiring associates, tell them you'll teach them all that you know, and also require of them what's needed to be successful. In fact, you'll teach, empower, and push them to break one of your clinic records. I set a goal to teach all my associates to surpass my own numbers.

4. Put together one or two hours of weekly training for your associate.

5. Sixty days prior to your next vacation, meet with your team and pick out two or three clinic records to break (high reexams? most new patients on a Thursday morning?). Now help your associate lead your staff to break the records and bring a huge win for everyone—especially you.

50

Developing Successful Associates

"Well, Noel," said the physician, "you need a two-level vertebrae fusion—5-6C and 6-7C. We can do that now, or a year from now when you're screaming in pain."

How's that for a report of findings? I knew it would be a cold day in hell before I'd let him cut on me. I've seen the human debris that many of those surgeries create. No thanks.

I drove away from the surgeon's office depressed and wondering what in the world I'd do. Just a couple of months earlier, I was personally seeing over 420 chiropractic visits a week, and my clinic was happily churning away at 650 to 720 weekly visits. But that was before an accident cost me 75 percent of the strength in my right arm. I couldn't practice anymore, and I was in constant, severe, radiating pain. I knew my life was going to change; I just didn't know how.

I didn't have the surgery. Instead, I designed a chiropractic and physical therapy program and adhered to it religiously. Years later,

I've completely rehabbed and have no strength or neurological deficits whatsoever. Thank you, chiropractic.

Want to know what happened to my practice? We went from seven hundred visits a week with me *working in* the practice to seeing over two thousand visits a week with me *working on* the practice. In fact, I was on a two-week vacation when I got word that for the first time we had seen more than two thousand patients in a week—and I was seven thousand miles away and under eighty feet of water.

So how did I turn a career-ending injury into the best job in the world—developing successful associates?

To start, I needed a good, hard look at three things.

First, how the business part of my practice was working. After looking at the business, I knew I needed better systems and more consistent training. Remember, *you get what you inspect, not what you expect.* Better training cut my stress in half and increased my profit margin significantly.

Second, how to get lots and lots of new patients from internal and external marketing. I had been unconsciously good at referrals and marketing for years. Now I intentionally took what I knew and packaged it up to teach to my DCs. This worked so well that we opened a new clinic with 161 new patients the first month—without me even being there.

Third, how to attract and develop top-notch chiropractors. If my practice had a prayer of going on without me, this was and is my most important project.

The following are my First Seven Essential Steps for Developing Successful Associates:

1. ***Get a clear picture of the benefits.*** Here's my short list of benefits:

   (a) *Help more people:* You can double or triple the number of people served by chiropractic in your community with associates. Plus, most of the DCs you train will be grateful for the help. Many of my former associates are still good friends.

(b) *Have more fun*: It's fun to teach good systems that you know work, then watch someone else succeed and reach their goals.

(c) *Be more successful*: You can serve more patients, and your associates are profitable and well-paid in as little as sixty days. Plus, I increased my free time and income.

2. **Get a crystal-clear picture of who to pick and how to develop them.**

The first thing I'll ask in an interview is "What do you want to be doing in five years?" If their goals don't match mine, I don't hire them. As for training, my motto is "two hours a week, times fifty weeks a year, equals a million-dollar practice." I provide consistent training in all areas of success.

I can hear some of you saying, "I don't have the time for that!" Do you have time to have a rotten associate? My two hours a week in training has given me doctors and staff who run $500,000 to $1,000,000 practices for me with no other time required. *Not training correctly is the biggest mistake doctors make with associates.*

3. **Handle the new patient problem.** Great DCs who can't get new patients fail. Average DCs who know how to get new patients succeed. Add training on how to get new patients, and start your associate with external marketing *their very first day on the job.*

4. **Build what the associate really wants.** Associates want to be successful. I truly care about my associates' success, and I've designed a path they can follow that leads them to great skills and an opportunity for owning their own practice.

5. ***Build in protection.*** You have an extremely valuable asset
   in your practice. To protect it, you'll need a well-thought-
   out, well-written contract that's reviewed and modified by an
   attorney in your state or province. Never hire anyone without
   one.

6. ***Plan on hard work and problems.*** I'd be lying if I told you I
   didn't work hard at this. But once I assembled the systems,
   templates, and protocols, the whole thing almost ran itself.

7. ***Assemble a mastermind group of other DCs who are developing successful associates.*** Recently, my mastermind group
   met in Hawaii to brainstorm, instruct each other, and improve our skills. We had a blast. This type of group is an
   absolute must.

These seven steps can be the start to replicating your success in
others and developing successful associates.

51

The Most Important Question You'll Ever Ask Your Associate

Before you hire a chiropractor to join your practice, it's critical to find out if your potential associate's goals are compatible with yours.

Needing a paycheck and being attracted to an energetic and well-run practice are understandable reasons that might drive someone to apply for the position. And your prospective associate may *forget* or even hide other strong desires in order to land the job and work for you.

However, after a few short days or weeks, when they discover that building a great practice is hard work, they may be asking themselves, "Why in the world am I doing this?" Why, indeed. Their immediate answer needs to be "because my long-term professional and personal goals are furthered greatly in my associate-ship."

If not, and your associate holds different long-term professional and personal goals, you just might get a letter on your desk some Monday morning explaining how the two of you weren't a "good fit," and promising to mail the office keys back by the end of the week.

How can you know ahead of time if this will happen?

The most important fit between a clinic director and associate is in the area of long-term goals. I can't count the times I've taught that *shared goals build unity*, and the examples are too numerous to even mention. If you know and are pursuing your goals, and those goals do not support your associate's goals, a split is inevitable.

How do we steer clear of this mistake? Become an expert at discerning your employee's long-term goals.

In your interview, ask the candidate, "What do you want to be doing in five years?" Listen carefully to what they tell you. If they are strongly committed to goals that are consistent with yours, and you're willing to help them reach those goals, you have a good chance of arriving there together.

Show real interest in their answers by asking follow-up questions like "Why is that important?" and "How long have you thought that?" Then look for their eyes to light up when they answer.

Beware of the person who's passionate about a totally different practice model than you have. I get nervous when someone tells me they just want to focus on a specific patient group (like only kids or athletes). Or if they want to "spend a lot of time with their patients to really get to know them." Both of these answers signal to me a weak self-image and poor understanding of chiropractic.

I'm even more leery of the person without any goals or, my least favorite, the candidate who tells you they want to be "cutting back" in five years. Don't even get me started on that guy.

In short, become an expert on reading what a potential associate really wants and why they are in chiropractic in the first place *before* you make them an offer.

After all, isn't it your desire to work shoulder to shoulder with an associate who loves the things you love? Of course it is. It takes a young doctor some time to really understand the process you're committed to taking them through, but don't make the potentially fatal error of failing to find out their long-term professional goals.

52

Keys to Win-Win Associate Development

A doctor approached me at a seminar, white as a sheet. "I just got off the phone. All of my associates in all three offices have just moved my practices down the street, and my attorney says my contract's worthless."

After I asked a few questions and then told him what I'd do, he said, "Boy, I wish I'd talked to you first."

Boy, did he ever.

Every month I get calls from doctors who end up saying, "Boy, I wish I'd talked to you first." Sometimes it's a minor irritation, but occasionally it's a full-scale train wreck that's already cost tens—if not hundreds—of thousands of dollars and too many sleepless nights.

With few exceptions, the biggest problems have to do with associates.

In almost every case, one or more of what I call the Seven Keys to Win-Win Associate Development were ignored or poorly done.

These keys are also signposts or guides that warn of danger. They'll help you avoid becoming one of the "Boy, I wish I'd talked to you first" crowd.

Some of the keys will seem basic, even simple, but in my opinion, the careful execution of these seven steps, in sequence, has saved the day more times than I can count.

Here are the keys:

1. Have a clear picture of the benefits.

I like to look at a win-win relationship with an associate as having the following four benefits:

- **Help:** If you don't need help, don't hire an associate. Associates are only useful and profitable for those clinic directors who really need assistance seeing patients and marketing.
- **Freedom:** It's great to have a clinic that functions at, or close to, capacity without you. You can leave the office knowing that your associate can reach and actually beat your best-ever numbers. (Don't turn the office over to an associate on their first day on the job, but after training, you can leave the office and return to a newly set and meaningful record.)
- **Profit:** Done my Win-Win Associate Development way, both you and your associate will profit early (within sixty or ninety days) and every month after that. Your associate may buy also buy their practice—I've sold ten now—and may buy your practice as well. It's called building a buyer.
- **Developing great doctors:** There's a special satisfaction that comes with helping doctors reach their potential. Both mentor and mentee embracing a common goal in a win-win commitment—each to the other's success—is hard but rewarding work.

2. Know the who, what, and how.

Who: Some associates are diamonds in the rough, while others really don't want to do what's required to be successful. I ask each associate what they want to be doing in five years. If the person's goals match mine, there's a chance things might work.

What: It's essential to lay out the first steps to keep everyone on the same track. I lay out a plan to take my associates to a $100,000 annual income and then work backwards through the steps. It's an attractive goal for the associate and gets everyone behind the training and challenges that are just ahead.

How: Most Monday nights for the last twenty-five years have found me training my associates. Ask yourself if your associate program is worth two hours, one night a week. It's important to set aside intentional time to train on marketing, new patient assisting, and procedures and scripts for Day One and Day Two.

3. Tackle the new patient problem.

The single biggest reason chiropractors fail is that they don't produce enough new patients. So introduce your associates to marketing as soon as possible. Clinic directors who end up feeding their new patients to the associate make a huge mistake.

4. Do an associate business plan before you hire.

Calculate how many visits a new associate will need to do on patients they recruit for you in order to break even on your investment, and coach them to that goal ASAP. My associates are typically profitable in sixty to ninety days.

5. Build in protection.

You're the one with the most to lose. You have worked on your practice for ten, fifteen, or maybe even more than twenty-five years.

You've trained the staff, built a good name in the community, and have a valuable asset. That investment needs protecting. Get a good contract that protects your practice, written in your state by a top attorney.

6. Build what the associate really wants.

If you've chosen well, your associate wants to learn, learn, and learn. I work to give my doctors a million-dollar education. In return, I get great associates who actually stay longer because I'm committed to training them and seeing them earn well.

7. Plan on hard work and problems.

Even a good associate is your most challenging hire. You'll need to be sharp and ready to deal with things that are more complicated than CA issues. You can have a great series of associates who are no challenge at all—and then the difficult one shows up. What will you do?

Plan ahead. I'm always reading a new coaching or management book designed to give me the best information on leading my associates to a successful future.

53

Avoiding the Associate Train Wreck

Every week, good and smart chiropractors tell me their associate train wreck stories. The following are four of the most common and costly mistakes and will show you what a strong associate program looks like done right.

Associate Mistake #1: Failure to Follow a Win-Win Associate Recipe

Whether it's putting together Ikea furniture or Grandma's meatloaf, there's a ton that can go wrong if you don't follow instructions or recipes. Great artists of every kind are moved by inspiration, but they also follow proven paths to bring their creations into reality. Each one discovered their process through painful, tedious trial and error, or they shortcut the learning time by learning from another.

With associates, there is a recipe for producing helpful, profitable, and content members of the team. If you miss even one of the critical steps, you may have to scrap your assembly and start all over again.

Throughout the entire process of interviewing, hiring, and bringing an associate into your clinic culture, up to profit, and then to full production, there are correct steps to take. Each one of those steps leads to another, is logical, keeps you in control, and most importantly, works for both director and associate.

The wrong way is to hope in blind luck. Throwing the latest candidate against the wall, hoping they stick, seldom if ever works and can be damaging to the practice and not worth the risk. Instead, get the best recipe(s) you can. A great associate is worth the search.

Done Right: Dr. Brian Morris of Ohio did everything wrong the first time he hired an associate, and he ended up with more stress and less money. This time he followed a successful recipe, selected the right person (shared goals), and trained them in his technique and procedures.

Result: Dr. Morris was able to take two week-long vacations without a hitch. In fact, things are working so well, Dr. Morris has hired a second associate.

Associate Mistake #2: Failure to Do an Associate Business Plan

Most associateships end badly because the clinic owner did not think about the business implications of hiring an associate. Don't rush to hire an associate just because you're busy; I can't tell you the number of clinic owners I've talked to who are pulling their hair out because they failed to do an associate business plan and now the business part of having an associate is not working because the associate costs more money than they produce. In addition, the associate is taking a portion of the clinic owner's new patients, and the clinic owner is experiencing a drop in gross and net income.

When doing an associate business plan, ask yourself the following questions:

- How many new patients does my associate need to generate to pay for themselves?
- How many patient visits per week does my associate need to see to pay for themselves?
- What additional services can the associate do for me to generate additional income to cover their salary and related expenses?

Done Right: Dr. Leah Meadows of Washington calculated her associate could collect more than his base salary in his first month because of a unique marketing opportunity. She was right, and because of a good business plan with sharp marketing, her associate never cost the clinic money he hadn't collected first.

Result: That associate ended up in bonus in just five months. Everyone wins!

Associate Mistake #3: Failure to Solve the New Patient Problem Beforehand

You built your practice over five or twenty years, and now you decide you need an associate to help you care for all the people you've acquired over that time.

The associate comes in, and only then do you notice that your practice volume was mainly because of a high patient visit average. You aren't generating enough new patients for two doctors. In just a few months, you notice that the practice is no longer busy, but you have an extra salary to pay, plus everybody is getting tense and irritable.

I have been on the phone with very bright doctors who were scratching their heads and wondering where half their net income went. These doctors did not solve the new patient problem beforehand.

This is a big error, and it's expensive.

To correct that error, let's start with a few questions: *Do you have new patient marketing opportunities that you have to pass on because you're too busy? Can you think of two or three events or programs you could do each week if you had any extra time?* If you can say an honest yes, you have a chance of solving the new patient problem beforehand.

Why is this important? Because you want your associate to succeed, pull their own weight, and learn to build their own practice rather than share yours. More associates are harmed by clinic owners not training them (and requiring they learn) to generate their own new patients than anything I know. The associate ends up "new patient disabled."

Done Right: Dr. Jeff Schels of Texas trained his associate how to produce his own new patients "fresh out of the egg," and now his associate has built a practice of 200+ patient visits a week and continues to produce his own new patients.

Result: Dr. Schels has developed (trained, coached, and mentored) an associate who has earned a special long-term associate employment arrangement. Now Jeff's only worry is keeping just a little bit ahead of his associate.

Associate Mistake #4: Failure to Have the Associate's Best Interest at Heart

Who are the people who bring out the best in you? I'm just guessing, but no matter how long or short a list you come up with, I bet these people have your best interest at heart. It's so simple: **we give our best efforts for the people we know want to see us succeed.**

When developing associates, you need to have their successful development at the top of your list. The associate needs to know that you're just as interested in their success as you are your own.

Some clinic directors look at associates as "exam and X-ray dogs" or "drones" who just do what they are told to do. This does not inspire loyalty or above-and-beyond effort on your associate's part.

One of the ways to demonstrate that you have the associate's best interest at heart, and help your associate business plan at the same time, is to take time out of your schedule to train your doctor.

Share the knowledge that you've accumulated over the years. Remember, so much of the information you take for granted today came at a price over years. When you spend time training your associate, they know that you care. The right associate will take that to heart and give you their best efforts.

Done Right: Imagine that your son or daughter was just getting out of chiropractic college, but not practicing with you. What would you want their clinic director to do? Offer them a contract with a pay structure where they could make great money if they earned it? Train and teach them? Require your kid to give the best they have? Hold them accountable? Praise and reward good work?

Result: I'm a dad, so I know what your answers were. My older boy works for my best friend in a training program just like that. Both my son and I are thrilled.

54

Building and Selling Satellite Practices

Over the years, I've built and sold ten satellite practices. I've trained others who've done between three and a dozen successful satellite sales. I truly love the process and have developed a low-stress formula that I'll share with you now.

In short, I hire and train associates who want to be clinic owners. When an associate qualifies for their own clinic, we carefully plan and build up the business of the satellite to such a successful level that the associate practically runs to me with a check in hand, eager to buy the practice.

The DC gets training and then a great practice. I get a check. It's a perfect win-win.

However, that all begs many important questions that require precise and important answers.

How do you know you have the right associate?

You screen for them. By now, you know I love spinal screenings, and not just because they produce thousands of new patients over decades. I also like the process and know how to make it fun.

I find associates the same way. I screen for them.

1. My ads screen for the doctor who's looking for a job *now* but wants to be an owner someday.
2. My interview questions check long-term goals and compatibility.
3. My tests check entrepreneurial aptitude.
4. My employment offer includes a detailed explanation of the entire process from associate to owner, including the price of the future satellite. I also include a list of my former associates who are now clinic owners and encourage the doctor to get in touch and ask questions about the process.

I need the associate to see that accepting my offer is truly the best option for both of us. It must be win-win. I've actually pushed qualified applicants in another direction. Why? There's a lot of hard work involved in building a practice, and I don't want anyone to regret their decision—including me. When a sharp, young DC's *other* choice was to own their parent's practice for free, guess where I sent that doctor. ("Go home, kid.")

How do associates qualify for their own clinic?

Once my carefully chosen associate is hired, I train the person in every aspect of building a practice, starting with new patient marketing.

My associates start external marketing on their first day on the job, and that's not hyperbole. They're instructed to show up with their screening scripts memorized word-for-word and perfect. Then they go out with another associate, marketing CA, or me to do a spinal screening.

After that, they're required to produce two to three events per week to build their marketing skills and their practice. If they can't do it, they don't qualify. It's just that simple.

The "mother ship" clinic is the only place to test associates to see if they're ready for their own office. That's also where I train clinic skills and patient management. The right person builds quickly.

How do you plan out the satellite practice?

My first consideration in planning a new office is identifying where the new patients will be. As an example, I strategically picked a space in a seventy-six-story office building that was connected to two other tall office towers. The lunch traffic went right by my office and screening station. We were at 186 fee-for-service visits a week in just three months.

Honestly, I won't sign a lease for a satellite unless the path to a successful build and sale is crystal clear to both the associate and me.

How do you build the satellite practice?

Remember how qualified associates get qualified? They have to be good at marketing. Part of the process of planning out the new satellite office is designing the marketing, so we build everything to the "I can't wait to buy my office!" level right from the beginning.

By this point, the associate has proven their ability to administrate my systems under my direction while in the mother ship. The DC ends up doing most of the work of launching the satellite, and that constitutes their training to be an owner.

Watching and working alongside associates as they work to qualify and then as they serve as the project manager for the satellite will tell you if they're worth the risk.

How do you sell the satellite practice?

Only for cash, so think about your buyer. An important filter for selecting the right associate is his or her credit. Financial train wrecks make terrible associates and never qualify as practice buyers. People who don't manage their own finances well don't take responsibility and often are blamers. Guess who they're going to blame for their problems? You.

Of course, there are literally dozens of other questions and answers, but this is the outline of the journey.

Now, I have some questions for you. Do you love the way your office works? Do you think it's a shame there's only one like it? You might be ready to consider helping a strong associate into his or her own practice.

55

Are Your Shareholders Happy?

Have you ever noticed how a new perspective or way of thinking about things can really make a job easier? Decades ago, I read several books from Ken Blanchard's *One-Minute Manager* series, and his systems revolutionized my management style and skills. Seth Godin's book *The Dip* was also incredibly helpful for developing associates.

There are dozens of these books in the business or personal development section at any bookstore. They provide new vantage points, and, typically with only about one hundred pages, can be read in an hour or two. You'll find your head buzzing with new and useful ideas to help your practice.

Many of my own best ideas have bubbled up in my brain when I was reading someone else's best ideas. This type of cerebral synergy is a great byproduct of these small and easily readable gems. I'm always looking for the next one, so if you have "the perfect book," please email me the title at noel@myfivestar.com.

My all-time favorite perspective changer is The *E-Myth Revisited* by Michael Gerber. Subsequent books on the same theme, such as The *E-Myth Physician*, have been disappointing, but *Revisited* continues to inspire me as a never-ending source of usable ideas. I have three well-worn, written-in, yellow-highlighted copies that I *revisit* frequently.

It's in chapter fourteen of Gerber's masterpiece that I found the seed for this idea. I call it the Shareholder-Employee concept.

Here's the idea: When thinking about our chiropractic practices, instead of the common, arrogant "lord of all we survey, where our word is law" perspective that many business owners have, chiropractors should take this position:

We are all employees, accountable to the shareholders.

Shareholders have invested in your company with the expectation of making a profit. The employees must always ask, "Are our shareholders getting their money's worth?"

I use this measuring stick regularly. Granted, as the business owner, I'm also the shareholder here, but the game has worked well for me in more ways than one.

Let me explain.

Here's the short list I review to see if the shareholders should be happy.

1. **Am I sharing the vision for where I'm taking the practice with my staff and patients?** The shareholders expect me to know where I'm going and to build a following. How can I do that unless I share where we're headed?

2. **Is my work consistent with my vision?** *Consistent* is the key word here. Can staff and patients count on me to do what I promise?

3. **Am I getting my projects done on time?** *Just getting the work done* may sound old-fashioned, but business owners without oversight frequently fall down in the area of accountability.

4. **Am I running clinic hours and patient care on time?** It's amazing how many offices don't grow because the doctor is undisciplined and takes too much of the wrong time with patients.

5. **Am I training my team to produce their best?** Are my front desk assistants, marketing assistants, and account managers all getting the training they need?

"The lord of all they survey" may not feel like being subjected to this line of questioning. "Who owns this place, anyway? I can do what I want!" That's true, but if your goals are different than the shareholders, maybe we've found a problem, and it's you who needs to change.

I remember an associate grousing about how my lead CA ran my clinic. "She pushes *everyone* around," he told me. His emphasis on *everyone* was for me, because I let her direct me and he thought that was terrible.

I responded, "Claudine does exactly what I want her to do. We both work for the goals of Sound Chiropractic. And she can move more than six hundred people through the office by herself and still leave, with her work done, by 6:10 every night."

The shareholders loved her.

There's a huge advantage to leading the team as an employee instead of the boss. Several times a week I have a conversation with a staff member where I use the statement "I work for the goals of Sound Chiropractic. My work is subject to review just like yours." This introduces fairness, builds unity, and keeps me on my toes.

Granted, I lead Sound Chiropractic's goal-setting meetings. I have authority to direct the process where I want it to go, but what

I want is for the other shareholders to also be happy with the goals
we set.

There are a number of things shareholders are looking at and
have a right to expect from me, like getting to the office early,
finishing chart notes on time, firing a staff person who refuses
to take the goals of the organization seriously, or completing any
other distasteful or boring aspect of the job. I get the best work
from *me* when I ask myself what the shareholders want.

A young associate told me he admired my management skill.
"Please teach me how to manage people like you do."

Here's what I told him: "The best managers are the best leaders,
and the best leaders do their job like they're killing snakes. Do your
job like your life depends on it. Imagine that important people
who you respect—we'll call them your shareholders—are counting
on you. Make them as happy as you can, and you'll be the leader
you want to be and well on your road to being a great manager."

56

Dr. Elliot's Story

Dr. Danielle Elliot was a great chiropractor with a strong chiropractic philosophy. She was hardworking and personable and loved meeting people. She met her first chiropractor at age eight, and that doctor greatly helped with her food allergies.

So why couldn't she get her struggling practice off the ground? She seemed to lose patients as fast as she got them. She was stumped.

She had a small but great office, a faithful CA, and a few patients who were crazy about her. But week after week, month after month, she had the same low numbers. After she covered expenses and student loans, she was barely scraping by. "I didn't spend $200,000 on chiropractic school for this."

Occasionally, she thought the practice was taking off, but then it would stall out and crash again, leaving her discouraged and needing to crawl back slowly. It was exhausting.

Dr. Elliot was chatting with an old classmate, Dr. Amanda McLain, at a homecoming reception. She could hardly believe what she heard.

Even though she graduated a year later than Danielle, Dr. McLain was seeing three times the patients, making three times the money, and by the sound of things, feeling a fraction of the stress. She was so busy, she said, she was considering hiring an associate.

"Uh, my experience is a little different than yours," Danielle said, grimacing. She thought, Amanda's in a smaller town, and she's not the outgoing people person I am, yet she's killing it. What's she doing differently? Okay, swallow the pride and just ask.

"Amanda, you see three times the people I do, and it sounds like it's easy for you. How do you do that?"

Dr. McLain wasn't the least bit condescending; in fact, she was just the opposite.

"Danielle, I was really blessed after graduation to be an associate in a great clinic that had so many of these things figured out for me. Now that I'm on my own, I understand how powerful they were. Why don't you come to my office for a half day and see for yourself? Then we'll have lunch, okay?"

Danielle readily agreed. Not wanting to be late, she arrived on the day of the meeting much too early and was surprised to see the office lights on and movement inside a full forty-five minutes before patients arrived. She went in.

"Morning! Am I late?"

"Come in, Dr. Elliot! You're right on time. Let me introduce you to the team." Amanda introduced her to two smiling, well-groomed, uniformed CAs, who greeted her courteously.

"We're getting ready for the day in our morning huddle," she explained. "Kristi's going to lead that now."

Kristi, the front desk CA, reviewed the schedule, told Dr. McLain where the tight spots were, and explained exactly what everyone needed to do to stay on time.

Amanda complimented each CA on a specific win from the day before, and Jenny, the other CA, read a short patient testimony just posted online.

When the meeting broke, Danielle said, "Wow, this is so organized. Do you do that every morning?"

"Every!" Dr. McLain smiled.

"Your report of findings is here, Doctor." Kristi joined them and indicated a happy-looking patient who'd just come in.

"Jason, do you mind if Dr. Elliot joins us this morning?"

"Not at all, Doc."

What Danielle saw was impressive. Amanda took just ten minutes to frame the working relationship, care goals, problem, care schedule, appointments, and financial solution. It was so smooth, so effortless. When she was done, she rang for Jenny.

"Jason, Jenny will help you with the finances and your appointments. Then she'll bring you to me for your first adjustment." Jenny smiled as she shook Jason's hand.

Danielle's head was swimming. It was all so professional!

Both doctors moved to the adjustment area, where patients were placed on three tables. Dr. McLain said a cheerful "Hi, guys!" to the three men lying face down and immediately went to work.

Danielle watched how relaxed Amanda was as she moved from patient to patient, expertly adjusting, instructing, and handling questions in courteous, short answers, but leaving no question about who was in charge and what would happen next.

When she was done, the patients made their way to unattended therapy. Dr. Elliot was impressed with how easy it felt. It was almost as if patient care was choreographed.

"James, tell my friend Dr. Elliot how long it's been since your last migraine," said Amanda, and the patient smiled as together they recounted a dramatic transformation.

"I love hearing your story, James, and I know you tell everyone. Do you need another free consultation certificate? Here, take two. And I hear that today Jenny's going to help you do a Google review for us. Did you bring your smart phone? Cool. Jenny, James is ready for you. See you next week."

Danielle had her iPhone out, texting notes about what she'd seen that morning.

Kristi appeared in the adjusting area with the morning stats on a Post-it note. "Great morning, Doctor. Wait times were virtually nonexistent, with thirty-one regular, two new, and your early ROF. If your charts are done, you can head out to lunch."

Danielle was a little surprised by that comment. *Who was actually in charge here?*

"Up-to-date, as promised, and I'm hungry. How about you, Danielle?"

The deli was a two-minute walk away, and after ordering, Danielle said, "It's all so smooth, so low stress. It's such a contrast from what I'm doing."

"What did you notice?"

"Tons. I made a list.

1. **Arrive early.** "You're serious about your staff coming in forty-five minutes early and strategizing before you get busy. The morning went just like Kristi said it would."

   "Yes, we are. It's a real business, and I've trained Kristi to run the practice just the way I want her to."

2. **Take control of each case.** "In your ROF, you took complete control, and the patient loved it."

   "That starts on Day One, but if they're a chiropractic case, that's my job. My certainty inspires their confidence."

3. **Make financial plans and multiple appointments.** "Love how you handle money and appointments right up front. It was easy."

"It usually is. Remember, patients are giving you their best decisions in the first three days. They want to get well. That means they need the appointments and so need to pay. We provide easy solutions for both."

4. **Run on time.** "Even with my numbers, I run late and feel stressed. You were never behind."

"We train on a very precise script. My patients have learned to expect me to be focused on them and also to respect their time."

5. **Stimulate referrals.** "I love the way you use certificates for referrals. Do they work?"

"Half of my new patients come from those referral certificates."

6. **Get Internet reviews.** "Tell me about how you do Google reviews."

"People used to promise they'd review us online and rarely did. Now we ask for permission to help them. They dictate the review to Jenny, who types it into their own smartphone and uploads it. So easy."

7. **Work as a team.** "I may know, but tell me why Kristi tells you when you can go to lunch? What's that?"

"We're a team. If my charts aren't done, I let the team down and send the message I don't care about our goals. I give her the authority to enforce the standard."

"This morning's been amazing. You said you learned all this as an associate. How?"

"I worked with a great office, where the doctor took his goals seriously and made sure we did too. When I saw all the systems, I soaked them up like a sponge. But there's one other thing you don't see. I also work with a practice coach, who reviews my stats and points out new ideas all the time.

And the consulting group is great. I'm constantly picking up great ideas from other members and fine tuning what I do." Danielle nodded. She had a whole new perspective for what her chiropractic practice could be.

Conclusion: Your Best-Ever Year

Friend, client, and full-time wild man, Dr. Phil Kriss competes in Ironman triathlons. That's where you swim 2.4 miles, bike 112 miles, and then run a 26.2-mile marathon. At fifty, Phil just scored his personal best time of under 11:07, finishing alongside the pros who have big sponsor money.

He was elated. I'm in awe. Over fifty and he's doing his best ever.

If you ask how he did it, he'll explain a very detailed training regimen, along with the science behind the physiology and his personal race strategy. He'll give you a checklist of what he does. Then he lets you decide if you want to pay the same price to produce *your* best-ever results.

"It's not rocket science. You want to do it, or you don't," I've heard Phil say.

What a lead-in! In the last four years, almost 80 percent of our consulting clients did their best-ever years in practice. For new practices, that's easy to understand, but I'm talking about doctors in their fifties, sixties—even seventies!

Now you have the same checklist they do for producing your own **best year ever** in practice. So then it's up to you. As Phil said, "It's not rocket science. You want to do it, or you don't."

Here's to your best-ever year in practice.

1. **Fall in love with the process.** You know real love is a choice, right? Make the choice to fall in love with the challenge, the growth, the skill acquisition, and the battle.

2. **Fall in love with your office visit.** You're going to do a zillion of 'em. Plan and map out an on-purpose, fun, and clinically excellent few minutes of pure bliss "by design." Train every patient to participate in that type of appointment, and if the patient refuses, refer him or her out to someone else.

3. **Fall in love with your report of findings.** Do a great ROF, and patients will follow you to the ends of the earth. Be so clear, so concise, and so persuasive that they can hardly wait to hear your ROF (and do it so well that patients will give you a standing ovation).

4. **Fall in love with your marketing.** Doctors who know how to market get lots of new patients and do well in practice. Doctors who don't, struggle for a lifetime. Learn to market. Learn to build and maintain three internal and three external marketing programs simultaneously in your practice. Dedicate three to seven hours a week to being your own marketing director. (That tip alone is worth $100,000 a year.)

5. **Find and keep good people.** Hire, train, develop, and keep good people. Share your practice vision with your staff, and train them how to work in cooperation with that vision. We have a phrase at Five Star that goes "2 x 50 = $1,000,000." That means two hours a week in training for fifty weeks a year will build a million-dollar practice.

6. **Go back to the basics.** Every golf coach on the planet will tell you that if their students just practiced the basics regularly, they'd all improve. What do you think the pros do? We need to sit with CAs, colleagues, or coaches and refresh, relearn, and practice our scripts and procedures to a polish. Remember what worked, and then do it again.

7. **Time everything.** I don't mean every appointment every day, but enough to *really* know how long it takes you to do everything in the office. I think some of you will be horrified. "No, it didn't take me that long, did it?" Yes, it did, Doctor, and that's why patients don't want to schedule. Ask your CA. And speaking of CAs...

8. **Go to work for a sharp CA.** Train a strong CA on how an office should run, and then give them the whip. Learn phrases like "Where do I need to be next?" and "What do you need from me?" and "Yes, sir/ma'am!" You'll be in great shape in no time.

9. **Know your stats.** If you can't measure it, you can't control it. Record keepers are record breakers, so keep records. Measure new patients, returning patients, regular patients, services, receipts, patient visit averages, office visit averages, and case visit averages.

10. **Watch your money.** You can't save or grow without a budget, so start there. Be a penny pincher. Know your gross collections, your overhead, your AR. Know what happens to every penny you don't collect, and why.

11. **Watch your mouth.** Make a decision to talk to your patients only about chiropractic philosophy. With your staff, praise their technique, encourage patient testimonies, and remind them how much you love "right now."

12. **Get out of your comfort zone.** Not wanting to do something can be an excellent reason to do it. Your comfort zone wants you dead and buried!

13. **Create your own mastermind group to share your dreams and goals in safety.** This consists of other successful DCs and business people, as well as your coach.

You can start with just one thing from this list, or pick three, five, or all thirteen. Whatever you do, find a good coach who'll encourage you to give your best to get your best.

Here's to your success!

Acknowledgements

I was eager to dedicate *The Chiropractor's Guide* to my lovely wife, Kate, but I want to thank and acknowledge her here, as well. Kate's career as a bestselling novelist has been such an inspiration and encouragement to me. Her example, wise counsel, and willingness to help me have literally made this book possible.

I also want to thank and acknowledge my editor, Beth Jusino, who walked this rookie through each step of the process, encouraging and prodding me when needed.

I'm grateful for the many wonderful doctors and chiropractic assistants of Sound Chiropractic Centers who worked shoulder-to-shoulder with me over decades as I developed, tested, polished, and perfected the procedures, systems and programs in this book.

And finally, I'm grateful to chiropractic for giving me back my health so many times. It is a privilege to be a chiropractor, sharing the gift of health with others. Times without number I've been struck with realization how blessed I am to be a chiropractor working with chiropractors.

About the Author

Dr. Noel Lloyd decided to become a chiropractor at the age of eleven with his father's encouragement. He graduated from Palmer College of Chiropractic in 1971 and founded Sound Chiropractic Centers in his home state of Washington.

Dr. Lloyd now heads up Five Star Management and The New Patient Academy, supporting chiropractors around the world.

He lives in Seattle with his wife, Kate.